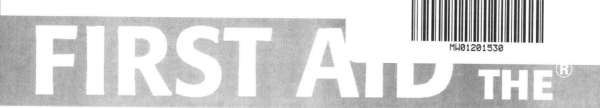

FIRST AID THE®

COMLEX
An Osteopathic Manipulative Medicine Review

Second Edition

ZACHARY NYE, DO
Resident
Department of Anesthesiology
Oregon Health and Science University
Portland, Oregon
OMM Fellow
Class of 2006
Department of Osteopathic Manipulative
    Medicine
Chicago College of Osteopathic Medicine
Downers Grove, Illinois

JOHN M. LAVELLE, DO
Resident
Department of Physical Medicine and
    Rehabilitation
Boston University
Boston, Massachusetts
OMM Fellow
Class of 2008
Department of Osteopathic Manipulative
    Medicine
Chicago College of Osteopathic Medicine
Downers Grove, Illinois

RACHEL LAVEN, DO
Resident
Department of Obstetrics and Gynecology
Lutheran General Hospital
Park Ridge, Illinois
OMM Fellow
Class of 2006
Department of Osteopathic Manipulative Medicine
Chicago College of Osteopathic Medicine
Downers Grove, Illinois

STOCKTON M. MAYER, DO
Resident
Department of Internal Medicine
University of Illinois Medical Center at Chicago
Chicago, Illinois
OMM Fellow
Class of 2008
Department of Osteopathic Manipulative Medicine
Chicago College of Osteopathic Medicine
Downers Grove, Illinois

Elise B. Halajian, Editor
OMM Fellow
Class of 2009
Midwestern University
Chicago College of Osteopathic Medicine
Downers Grove, Illinois

Stephen M. Huxley, Illustrator

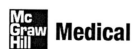 **Medical**

New York / Chicago / San Francisco / Lisbon / London / Madrid / Mexico City
Milan / New Delhi / San Juan / Seoul / Singapore / Sydney / Toronto

First Aid for the® COMLEX: An Osteopathic Manipulative Medicine Review: Second Edition

1 2 3 4 5 6 7 8 9 0   QPD/QPD   12 11 10 9 8

ISBN 978-0-07-160025-5
MHID 0-07-160025-6

NOTICE

This book was set in Electra LH by International Typesetting and Composition.
The editor was Catherine Johnson.
The production supervisor was Catherine Saggese.
Project management was provided by International Typesetting and Composition.
Quebecor World Dubuque was printer and binder.

This book is printed on acid-free paper.

To Dawn, Jonathan, Rebecca, Kirsten, Jack, Kathleen, and the rest of our friends, families, and teachers, without whom this venture would not have been possible. We also dedicate this book to the past, present, and future OMM Fellows.

CONTENTS

CONTRIBUTORS

Tamar Gibli

OMM Fellow
Class of 2009
Midwestern University
Chicago College of Osteopathic Medicine
Downers Grove, Illinois

Melissa Greer

OMM Fellow
Class of 2010
Midwestern University
Chicago College of Osteopathic Medicine
Downers Grove, Illinois

Kerri Kulovitz

OMM Fellow
Class of 2010
Midwestern University
Chicago College of Osteopathic Medicine
Downers Grove, Illinois

Melissa A. Novak, DO

Resident
North Memorial Medical Center Family Medicine Program
University of Minnesota
Minneapolis, Minnesota
OMM Fellow
Class of 2007
Midwestern University
Chicago College of Osteopathic Medicine
Downers Grove, Illinois

Dawn Nye, DO

Resident
Department of Anesthesiology
Oregon Health and Science University
Portland, Oregon
Class of 2006
Midwestern University
Chicago College of Osteopathic Medicine
Downers Grove, Illinois

Terry Pexton, DO

Resident
Department of Internal Medicine
Scripps Mercy Hospital
San Diego, California
OMM Fellow
Class of 2007
Midwestern University
Chicago College of Osteopathic Medicine
Downers Grove, Illinois

First Aid for the COMLEX: An Osteopathic Manipulative Medicine Review is a high-yield board review text of osteopathic manipulative medicine (OMM) for the Comprehensive Osteopathic Medical Licensing Examination (COMLEX) Steps 1, 2, and 3. Osteopathic concepts are taught in various frameworks across the country at different institutions. Please be assured that the information in this text was only collected from widely accepted osteopathic literature in order to include the majority of this information.

The focus of the text is to emphasize the material most commonly encountered on the COMLEX. That being noted, it must be understood there is no guarantee that this text covers every single osteopathic manipulative medicine question presented on the exam. Your feedback is strongly encouraged regarding the content of the review book in addition to how well prepared you felt for the OMM portion of the examination after using this text. Should you wish to share this feedback with the authors directly, you may do so by sending an email to: *firstaidforthecomlex@gmail.com.*

First Aid for the COMLEX: An Osteopathic Manipulative Medicine Review was designed to be used as a review guide for the OMM portion of the COMLEX. In no way is it meant to be used as an all-inclusive reference source. Therefore, please note that the authors take no responsibility for consequences of applications or interpretations of information within this text including, but not limited to technique descriptions.

ACKNOWLEDGMENTS

We would like to thank the many individuals who helped us write *First Aid for the COMLEX*. Our appreciation extends to Aaron Bruce, whose tireless efforts helped to initiate this process. For greatly contributing to this book we thank Terry Pexton. For additional contributions we thank Tamar Gibli, Kerri Kulovitz, Melissa Greer, Dawn Nye, and Melissa Novak. For taking the time to review our works, we thank Daniel Davison, DO, Mark McKeigue, DO, Charles Mok, Jr., DO, Kenneth Nelson, DO, Mark Robinson, DO, and Melicien Tettambel, DO. For use of the Yogatrek Center and endless support, we thank Ben and Joan Taylor. For current and future revisions, we are grateful to our editor, Elise Halajian. For last-minute phone calls, questions, and for always being available, we thank Marsha Loeb. And finally, we extend gratitude to our publishing editor, Catherine Johnson, for guiding us through these uncharted waters.

Guide to Efficient Examination Preparation

▶ Introduction

Introduction

First Aid for the COMLEX: An Osteopathic Manipulative Medicine Review is a high-yield board review text of osteopathic manipulative medicine (OMM) for the Comprehensive Osteopathic Medical Licensing Examination (COMLEX) Steps 1, 2, and 3.

There are five main sections in this text. The first section is comprised of a guide to efficient examination preparation. The second section provides an overview of various OMM technique modalities (specific technique descriptions are included later in the text). The third section looks at regional diagnosis and treatment, focusing on relevant anatomy and key diagnostic points. The fourth section contains a variety of high-yield tables for viscerosomatic/ Chapman reflexes, Jones' counterstrain tenderpoints, musculoskeletal tests, and noteworthy historical references. The fifth section involves an overview of commonly encountered techniques and includes brief descriptions and indications for each.

Information regarding OMM for clinical specialties (obstetrics and gynecology, pediatrics, the hospitalized patient, cardiology, gastroenterology, etc) is included in the second section. These topics are particularly useful when reviewing for board examinations because a large majority of OMM questions found in the COMLEX focus on specific patient cases and clinical vignettes.

Aside from the high-yield review of osteopathic manipulation concepts, students will also find information regarding the COMLEX performance evaluation (PE). Particular emphasis is placed on the role of OMM in the examination and the various OMM techniques permitted during the examination.

The vast differences in terminology and techniques used between various osteopathic colleges make creating an osteopathic review text difficult. The fifth section in this book attempts to describe techniques *commonly* included in board examination questions. The technique descriptions provide information about the techniques relevant to the COMLEX written examination (ie, indications, patient positioning, and the predominant final corrective force) and are not meant to replace technique manuals at specific osteopathic colleges. Although each technique described in this book is referenced from a major osteopathic source, they are not recommended for use in passing practical examinations.

Description of the COMLEX

The COMLEX is designed to assess both medical knowledge and clinical skills. In order to accomplish this, the National Board of Osteopathic Medical Examiners (NBOME) has developed an overall blueprint. This general blueprint is used for each step of the COMLEX examination (see Table 1-1); however, the content of each examination is tailored to the knowledge level of the test taker. The examination covers two main areas. The first (Dimension I) is known as *the clinical presentation*. This involves health topics frequently encountered by general practice osteopathic physicians. The second area (Dimension II) is known as *the physician task*. This involves the decision-making abilities that physicians use to problem-solve a particular medical issue. Osteopathic manipulative techniques (OMT) topics are dispersed throughout this blueprint, covering all areas within these two sections.

4

TABLE 1-1. The COMLEX Examination Blueprint

Dimension I: Patient Presentation

LEVEL 1, LEVEL 2-CE, LEVEL 3

Asymptomatic and general symptoms	8%-16%
Symptoms and disorders of digestion and metabolism	4%-10%
Symptoms and disorders of sensory alternations	28%-38%
Symptoms and disorders of motor alternations	6%-12%
Symptoms and disorders related to human sexuality and urination	3%-8%
Symptoms and disorders of respiration and circulation	8%-16%
Symptoms and disorders of thermoregulation	2%-6%
Symptoms and disorders of the tissues and trauma	8%-16%
Symptoms and disorders of human development	3%-8%

Dimension II: Physician Tasks

	LEVEL 1	LEVEL 2-CE	LEVEL 3
Health promotion and disease prevention	1%-5%	15%-20%	15%-20%
History and physical	5%-15%	30%-40%	10%-20%
Diagnostic technologies	1%-5%	10%-20%	15%-25%
Management	2%-7%	10%-20%	25%-40%
Scientific understanding of mechanisms	70%-85%	5%-15%	5%-10%
Health-care delivery	1%-3%	5%-10%	5%-10%

CE, cognitive evaluation.

LEVEL 1

COMLEX Level 1 is created using the COMLEX examination blueprint. The emphasis of this examination is placed on utilizing knowledge of basic science, in the areas of anatomy, behavioral science, biochemistry, microbiology, osteopathic principles, pathology, pharmacology, and physiology.

LEVEL 2

COMLEX Level 2-cognitive evaluation (CE) is also created using the COMLEX-USA blueprint; however, there is greater emphasis placed on topics found in the second area of the blueprint (Dimension II). These topics involve arriving at medical diagnoses using history and physical (H&P) examination information. Disciplines in this examination include emergency medicine, family medicine, internal medicine, obstetrics and gynecology, osteopathic principles, pediatrics, psychiatry, and surgery.

LEVEL 3

As with Levels 1 and 2, Level 3 is created using the COMLEX-USA blueprint. In this examination, the emphasis is shifted toward patient management. The test requires the examinee to solve the types of medical problems, a general practice osteopathic physician might encounter. The disciplines involved in the examination are the same as those found in Level 2.

In 1995, the NBOME changed the delivery method of the COMLEX from a 2-day written examination containing 750 questions to a 1-day computer-based examination containing 400 questions. The last written examination available was the Level 1 examination in October 1995. The new computer-based examination is delivered throughout the year at more than 300 locations throughout the country.

The computer-based examination contains eight blocks of 50 questions each. Once the examinee has left a particular block, they may not return to that block and modify their answers. There are two types of breaks during the examination. After completion of sections two and six, there will be an optional 10-minute break. This break will count against the total time the examinee has to take the entire examination. After completion of block four, there will be an optional 40-minute lunch break. This time is not counted against the total time allotted to complete the examination. If the examinee returns to take block five after the 40 minutes have ended, any remaining time more than 40 minutes will count against the total time allowed to complete the examination.

Registration, payment, scheduling, canceling, rescheduling, and withdrawing are all completed through an online system. This system is also used to receive available testing dates and locations. For more information on registration, visit www.nbome.org.

Grading of the Examination

The number of correct items is converted to both a 3-digit and 2-digit score. The mean 3-digit score is 500, for all steps of the examination. The minimum score needed to pass Levels 1 and 2 is 400; for Level 3 the minimum passing score is 350. The standard deviation of the 3-digit score depends on the year in which the exam was taken. For example, the standard deviation for Level 1 from 2002 to 2005 was 79, for Level 2 from 2001 to 2005 was 73, for Level 3 from 2000 to 2005 was 120.

The minimum 2-digit score needed to pass is 75 for all levels of the examination. Like the 3-digit score, the standard deviation of the 2-digit score depends on the year in which the exam was taken. For Level 1, the standard deviation from 2002 to 2005 was 3.95; for Level 2, the standard deviation between 2001 and 2005 was 3.65; and for Level 3, the standard deviation from 2000 to 2005 was 4.00.

The number of examinees who pass or fail the test depends on their performance in the examination and is not determined prior. A passing score is based on the overall examination, not on specific areas. The COMLEX score report does however provide graphic information regarding how well a particular test taker performed on specific areas of the examination. Students can typically expect their scores 4 weeks after the examination. However, the scores cannot be released until a reasonable number of examinees have taken the given test. Therefore, examinees who take the test earlier may have to wait longer to receive their results.

OMT on the COMLEX

The NBOME incorporates OMT into roughly 20% of questions found on all three levels of the COMLEX. These questions are typically straightforward. Commonly, people omit studying for the OMT questions on the COMLEX thinking that OMT is not significantly represented. However, 20% is a significant portion. Therefore, mastering manipulative medicine concepts can greatly elevate one's overall score.

Many osteopathic medical institutions emphasize themes in their curriculums that are also emphasized on the COMLEX. The authors of this book recognize cranial, sacral, and viscerosomatic reflexes as three commonly encountered topics. Chapters and tables in the text dedicated to these areas of interest are vital to success on written board examinations.

There are two major question formats on the COMLEX: block questions and stand-alone questions. Stand-alone questions are individual questions with a one-question stem. Block questions start with a question stem followed by two to five questions pertaining to that stem. Some blocks are all OMT, meaning the question stem is related to an OMT case and each question pertaining to the stem asks OMT questions. Some blocks deal with a particular case and only one of the questions pertains to OMT. For example, the case may deal with a patient with appendicitis. Most of the questions will ask about appendicitis, with one question asking about where you would find a viscerosomatic response in this patient.

▶ PE EXAMINATION

The PE/clinical skills examination of the COMLEX-USA Level 2 is intended to assess the medical student's knowledge of focused physical examinations, as well as evaluate their interpersonal and communication skills. This is a requirement for all osteopathic medical students. Scheduling for this examination should be done as early as possible during the fourth year. Spots fill up very quickly and it is best to reserve a time early. As the testing date approaches, examinees should refer to the orientation guide for COMLEX-USA Level 2-PE on the NBOME Web site at www.nbome.org. A 27-minute informational program video on the Web site shows the actual testing center, the documents used throughout the test, and a few examples of mock examinations.

Outline of Examination

There are 12 clinical encounters involving standardized patients (SPs). Approximately 14 minutes are allotted to reading the doorway information sheet (patient's name, type of clinical setting, chief complaint, and vital signs), performing the H&P, and using any necessary OMT. The examination allows approximately 9 minutes for the completion of a subjective, objective, assessment, plan (SOAP) note. If the medical student finishes the encounter prior to the 14 minutes, they can begin writing the SOAP note. However, additional discussion or examination of the SP is prohibited.

Walk Through of Test Day

On the day of the examination, remember to dress professionally, wear a white coat, and bring a stethoscope. Aside from a pen, these are the only items permitted in the testing area itself. The NBOME recommends arriving at the testing center 30 minutes prior to the start of the examination. Be sure to leave ample travel time and account for travel delays to the testing center. Be aware that the clinical encounters do not begin for at least an hour and a half after arriving on-site.

Upon arrival, examinees will officially sign in and be photographed for security purposes. Examinees will then be led to a conference room, which will serve as the "home-base" throughout the day. Personal belongings are then placed into lockers and *may not be retrieved* until the examination has been completed. Any item potentially needed during the course of the day should be kept in the conference room and not placed in a locker.

The NBOME provides a 50-minute orientation consisting of a video presentation very similar to that found on the Web site and an oral presentation with accompanying PowerPoint. The orientation reviews many of the key points highlighted on the Web site and in the informational video. Following orientation, there is a 15- to 20-minute break during which examinees are permitted to familiarize themselves with the power tables and various instruments in the testing rooms. Examinees are also free to visit the restrooms at this time.

After the break has ended, examinees are led into the main testing facility. This room is the starting point for all clinical encounters and leads to each of the 12 testing rooms. The 12 clinical encounters are broken down into three sets of 4. A 30-minute break follows the first set of four patient encounters and a small meal is provided during this time. Examinees are permitted to bring food to the examination center, but refrigeration is not available. The authors of this book suggest bringing extra snacks in case box lunches are not sufficient. Following the second set of four patient encounters, a 15-minute break is given. An opportunity to complete an evaluation of the testing experience is provided after the third set of patient encounters. Examinees may leave the testing center upon completion of the evaluation.

Please note, the orientation and both examination breaks take place in the conference room. A proctor is present in the conference room at all times to monitor any discussion that may pertain to the examination because such discussion is strictly prohibited.

Content of Clinical Encounters and OMT

During the examination, the patient encounters incorporate a range of clinical settings and scenarios. From a family practice office to the emergency room, from pediatrics to geriatrics, and from a common cold to a specific musculoskeletal injury, examinees encounter a wide variety of cases. The patients may have specific complaints or they may be there for a well-patient visit. Well-patient visits may include prenatal visits, preparticipation sports, physicals, well-woman examinations, and school physicals. The patients are already gowned when an examinee enters the room. Female breast and pelvic examination and rectal or genitalia examination of either sex is absolutely prohibited during the examination. It is appropriate to suggest a rectal examination for occult blood in your plan, but such invasive examinations must not be performed.

Keep in mind that the overall goal of this examination is for the NBOME to assess whether students have developed the necessary skills required to begin a residency training program. The NBOME is not looking for the student who can best execute a manipulation technique. That noted, manipulation may not be necessary for all cases but osteopathic principles should be applied in *every* case. For example, be sure to palpate for viscerosomatic reflexes if the patient has gastrointestinal complaints. An examinee may choose not to perform OMT on the aforementioned patient, but documentation of the viscerosomatic reflexes demonstrates understanding of the osteopathic philosophy.

About 25% of the patient encounters involve OMT specifically. If OMT is warranted, it is recommended that only 3 to 4 minutes of the total encounter be spent on treatment. High velocity, low amplitude (HVLA) is the only type of manipulation that is absolutely prohibited during the examination. Soft tissue techniques, deep articulation, counterstrain, muscle energy, myofascial release, and facilitated positional release are examples of appropriate technique modalities examinees may choose to employ.

The following techniques may be useful during the COMLEX PE:

Chronic headaches—cervical soft tissue, "killer fingers" (myofascial release of the occipitoatlantal [OA] junction), cervical muscle energy, counterstrain of upper thoracics or rib tenderpoints that could be contributing to the headaches

Upper respiratory infection (URI)—myofascial release of thoracic inlet (to allow for increased lymphatic drainage from the head), sinus techniques (percussion of frontal and maxillary sinuses, inhibitory pressure of the three branches of the trigeminal nerve where they exit the cranium, nasal bone articulation), frontal lift, venous sinus drainage

Shoulder complaints (not caused by referred pain)—*treat the upper thoracics*, Spencer technique, counterstrain for anterior and posterior rib tenderpoints

Forearm/Wrist complaints—*treat the upper thoracics*, direct/indirect myofascial release of the forearm, carpal bone articulation, counterstrain of forearm tenderpoints

Cough/Shortness of breath (SOB)—thoracic soft tissue, myofascial release of the thoracic inlet, doming of the diaphragm, thoracic pump, rib raising

Chronic abdominal pain—thoracolumbar junction soft tissue or muscle energy, indirect techniques of the sacrum, rib raising

Low back pain—lumbar soft tissue, lumbar muscle energy, counterstrain of anterior lumbar tenderpoints (great place to start), psoas muscle energy, balanced ligamentous tension of the pelvis, indirect techniques of the sacrum, piriformis counterstrain, muscle energy of the ilium

Don't Forget To

- Introduce yourself upon entering the room.
- Wash your hands before examining the patient.
- Drape the patient appropriately during the physical examination.
- Perform OMT.

- Perform a structural examination if necessary.
- Check viscerosomatic reflexes.
- Perform a thorough neurological examination for cases involving radiculopathies.
- Appropriately close the encounter.

SOAP Note

The official SOAP note used during the examination can be accessed on the NBOME Web site. Examinees may not write on the official SOAP note during the patient encounters; however, it is acceptable to take notes on the doorway information sheet provided.

Like all SOAP notes, there is an area for the subjective and objective findings, an assessment, and a plan. Under the assessment section, five lines are provided for a differential diagnosis. One should attempt to supply five differentials. The first assessment written should be the most likely diagnosis. Five lines are also provided in the plan section. Items to include in the plan section may include antibiotic administration, necessary imaging studies, or more invasive diagnostic procedures (such as a rectal examination for occult blood or a colonoscopy). A signature is *not* necessary at the end of the SOAP note.

Scoring and Evaluation

The overall examination score will be reported as either pass or fail. Each encounter is evaluated based on two different domains. The first is the humanistic domain, which encompasses doctor–patient communication, interpersonal skills, and professionalism. The SPs are responsible for this part of the assessment and will fill out evaluations immediately following the encounter. The second domain is the biomedical/biomechanical domain. History and physical (H&P) skills, OMT principles and skills, and written SOAP notes are the basis for evaluation of this domain and will be rated by certified osteopathic physician examiners. An overall passing score for *both* domains is necessary to receive a pass for the COMLEX-USA Level 2-PE. Results are typically mailed out 10 to 12 weeks following the examination. This time frame may decrease as more and more osteopathic students take the examination.

Preparation for the Examination

Preparation for this examination takes place during the third and fourth years of medical school. Remember, the purpose of the examination is to ensure osteopathic medical students are adequately prepared to begin residency training. Communication with patients is just as important as writing a concise, informative SOAP note. Reviewing common medical problems and coming up with a differential diagnosis for each is an excellent preparatory exercise. When preparing for the OMT aspect of the examination, select a few techniques for each major body region and practice demonstrating them effectively and efficiently. Practice giving instructions in layman's terms so the SPs will understand you.

Finally, be sure to get a good night's rest before the examination. This means arriving in Philadelphia at a reasonable hour and getting settled at the hotel. Do not take the last flight out for the evening in case there are unforeseen problems with the flight. Most importantly, relax. Good luck!

OMT Fundamentals

- Somatic Dysfunction
- Overview of Techniques

CHAPTER 2

Somatic Dysfunction

Definition

- Impaired or altered function of related components of the somatic (body framework) system: skeletal, arthrodial, and myofascial structures; and related vascular, lymphatic, and neural elements

Characteristics

- A disturbance of the normal function of somatic structures
- Possesses the characteristics of TART
- Based on a neurophysiological phenomenon
- Can result in compromised health
- Responds appropriately to osteopathic manipulative techniques (OMT)

Think TART

- Tissue texture change
- Asymmetry
- Restriction of motion
- Tenderness

Components of TART

- **T**: Tissue texture change (see Table 2-1)
    - Palpable changes within the somatic tissues indicative of physiological dysfunction
    - Changes found in skin, fascia, and muscle
    - Acute versus chronic palpatory findings
- **A**: Asymmetry
    - A visual or palpatory difference in the bony or soft tissue alignment when compared to similar structures in the same area.
    - Example: A flexed spinal segment will produce a "speed bump" (spinous process will stick out farther) as compared to the other spinous processes in the same area.
- **R**: Restriction of motion
    - There will be a decreased range of motion in one or several directions of the affected joint.
    - Pay attention to the **quantity** of motion as well as the **quality** (end feel) of motion.
    - **Active motion** may be affected (ability of the patient to move the joint with his/her own force); this type of motion engages the **physiological barrier**.
    - **Passive motion** may be affected (motion produced by the force of the examiner exerted on the patient); this type of motion engages the **anatomical barrier**.
    - When somatic dysfunction is present, the **restrictive barrier** will be engaged (see Barrier Concept).
- **T**: Tenderness
    - This is a subjective finding upon palpation of the affected area; look at the patient for a change in facial expression.
    - The degree of pain reported is disproportionate to the amount of force applied by the examiner.
    - Response to pain is often involuntary.

Some schools discuss the components of STAR, substituting sensitivity for tenderness.

14

TABLE 2-1. Acute Versus Chronic Tissue Texture Change

ELEMENTS	ACUTE PALPATORY FINDINGS	CHRONIC PALPATORY FINDINGS
Texture	Boggy, rough	Thin, smooth
Temperature	Warm	Cool
Moisture	Increased	Dry
Tenderness	Significant	Present, but less significant
Edema	Present	Absent

Barrier Concept

- Describes the limitations of motion in one plane or several planes of motion.
- All motion has a **neutral point** for which the characteristics of motion (quantity and quality) are equal on both sides.
- Absence of somatic dysfunction (see Figure 2-1).
- Neutral point exists for which motion away from that point is equal toward either side.
- The active range of motion engages the **physiological barrier** (soft tissue restrictions).
- The passive range of motion engages the **anatomical barrier** (bony restrictions).
- Somatic dysfunction will alter the neutral point and change both characteristics of motion (see Figure 2-2).
- The neutral point shifts and now motion away from the original point is greater to one side than the other (in quality and quantity).
- This type of motion now engages the **restrictive barrier** (a functional restriction that limits the range of motion to even less than the physiological range of motion).
- The **pathological neutral** is formed, which brings back equal motion to both sides.
- A **pathological barrier** may also be present, which is a permanent restriction of joint motion caused by pathological changes of the somatic system (ie, osteoarthritis of the hip limits range of motion owing to joint space narrowing and bony changes).
- These concepts are important when determining what type of OMT to use.
- Direct techniques engage the restrictive barrier.
- Indirect techniques move toward the pathological neutral.

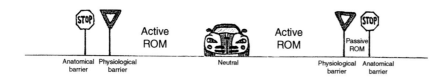

FIGURE 2-1. Range of motion in the absence of somatic dysfunction. The neutral point is exactly in the middle of the anatomical barriers.

15

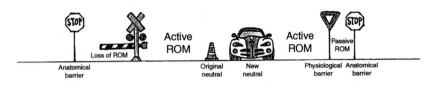

FIGURE 2-2. Range of motion in the presence of somatic dysfunction. The neutral point has been moved to accommodate for the lack of motion to one side.

If T3 is rotated to the right, the right transverse process is called the posterior component and the left transverse process is called the anterior component.

Concavity and convexity are used when discussing group curves (involving three or more vertebral segments), scoliosis, and certain cranial strain patterns.

Terminology of Spinal Motion and Somatic Dysfunction

- Vertebral segment—a single vertebra
- Vertebral unit—two adjacent vertebrae and all of their associated components (ie, arthrodial, ligamentous, muscular, neural, lymphatic)
- Group curve—consisting of at least three vertebral segments
- Posterior component
  - Describes the position of the vertebra when it is rotated
  - Typically referring to a prominent transverse process
- Anterior component
  - Also describes the position of the vertebra when it is rotated
  - Typically referring to the less prominent transverse process
  - This term is used less frequently
- Concavity
  - The inside of a curve (forms a CAVE)
  - The side to which sidebending occurs
- Convexity
  - The outside of a curve
  - The opposite side to which sidebending occurs
- Facilitation—the maintenance of a pool of neurons in a state of partial or subthreshold excitation
  - Refers to a spinal segment, which is being overloaded by input from somatic or visceral structures.
  - Takes the VS reflex to a new level.
  - The spinal segment remains hyperexcitable and leads to hypertonicity of the adjacent somatic structures.

Fryette's Principles

HISTORY

- H.H. Fryette, DO, first described the principles of physiological spinal motion in 1918. These principles describe typical spinal motion of a vertebral segment and groups of segments.
- These principles were applied only to typical vertebral segments—those which have articular facets and an intervertebral disc.

SIMPLE VERSUS COMPOUND MOTION

- Motion can be described as simple or compound.
- Simple—single motion of the spine that occurs in a sagittal plane about a transverse axis; either flexion or extension.
- Compound—motion that links multiple movements to each other.
- Addresses the sidebending and rotational components of a vertebral segment and its relationship with the simple motion of that same segment (flexion, extension, neutral).

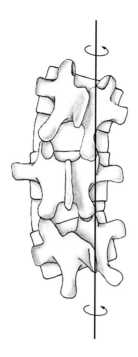

FIGURE 2-3. Fryette's Principle I. The spine is in neutral; rotation and sidebending occur to opposite sides.

FRYETTE'S PRINCIPLE I

(See Figure 2-3 and Table 2-2.)
- A subset of compound motion.
- Type I motion = neutral mechanics = group mechanics.
- Typically refers to a group curve in the thoracic and or lumbar regions of the spine.
- The neutral spine does not engage the articular facets.
- Rotation occurs into the convexity (which is produced by the sidebending).
- Maximum rotation will be at the apex of the group curve.

Fryette's Principle I: When the spine is in neutral (neither flexed nor extended), a group of vertebral segments will rotate and sidebend in opposite directions.

FRYETTE'S PRINCIPLE II

(See Figure 2-4 and Table 2-2.)
- A subset of compound motion.
- Type II motion = nonneutral mechanics = single segment mechanics.
- Typically refers to a single vertebral segment in the thoracic and or lumbar regions of the spine.
- The flexion or extension of the segment engages the articular facets.
- Rotation occurs to the side of the concavity (which is produced by the sidebending).

Fryette's Principle II: When a spinal segment is engaged in either flexion or extension, the same segment will rotate and sidebend in the same direction.

EXCEPTIONS TO THE RULE

- Occiput—rotates and sidebends to opposite sides
- Atlas—no significant sidebending component
- Sacrum—sidebending and rotation are coupled causing the sacrum to move about an oblique axis
- Cervical spine (C2-C7)—typically rotate and sidebend to the same side

---

Areas of the spine that do not follow Fryette's Principles I and II:

- Occiput
- Atlas
- Sacrum
- Cervical spine

TABLE 2-2. Comparison of Fryette's Principles

CHARACTERISTICS	PRINCIPLE I	PRINCIPLE II
Naming	Type I motion	Type II motion
	Neutral mechanics	Nonneutral mechanics
	Group mechanics	Single segment mechanics
Flexion/Extension component	Absent (neutral)	Present
Relationship of sidebending and rotation	Occurs to opposite sides	Occurs to the same side
Direction of rotation	Into the convexity	Into the concavity
Clinical findings	Lateral curve	Speed bumps—flexed segments causing the spinous process to stick out
		Pot holes—extended segments causing the spinous process to sink in

Typically movement in one plane will decrease movements in the other planes.

PHYSIOLOGICAL PRINCIPLE III (DEVELOPED AT A LATER POINT IN TIME)

Movement of a vertebral segment in any one plane will affect the motion of that same segment in other planes of motion.

Example: When setting up high velocity, low amplitude (HVLA) techniques, one plane of motion is engaged first (ie, sidebending in the frontal plane).

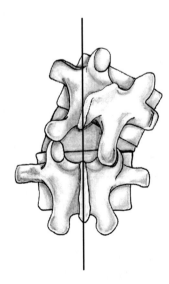

FIGURE 2-4. Fryette's Principle II. The spine is in nonneutral; rotation and sidebending occur to the same side.

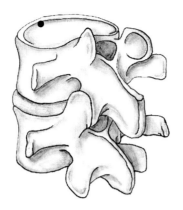

FIGURE 2-5. Frame of reference.

This will then decrease the amount of rotation possible in that same joint (within the transverse plane).

Naming Somatic Dysfunction

FRAME OF REFERENCE

- The anterior superior aspect of the vertebral body is used as the frame of reference (see Figure 2-5).
- Segmental motion is described by comparing the vertebral segment to the one below it.
- Example: The motion of T5 is described by using the anterior superior aspect of the vertebral body of T5 in relation to T6.
- Group mechanics (three or more segments) are described relative to the anatomical position.

Example: T2 to T7 as a group is sidebent right, rotated left in relation to the anatomical position.

WHO?

Which segment or group of segments has the dysfunction?

WHAT?

What will it do? This is usually how we write our findings.
  What won't it do? This is usually how we find our findings.

NAMING TYPE I SOMATIC DYSFUNCTION

- Identify the segment.
- Acknowledge that the segment is neutral.
- Describe the way in which the group moves more freely in rotation and sidebending (in opposite directions, of course).

Somatic dysfunction is most commonly named for the direction of FREER motion.

19

Example: T5NRRSL—identifies which segment has the somatic dysfunction, acknowledges the neutral (N) component of a Type I dysfunction, and describes the direction of rotation and sidebending to which it moves more freely.

NAMING TYPE II SOMATIC DYSFUNCTION

- Identify the segment.
- Acknowledge the flexion or extension component.
- Describe the way in which the segment moves more freely in rotation and sidebending (in the same direction, of course).

Example: L1FRSL—identifies which segment has the somatic dysfunction, acknowledges the flexion component of a Type II dysfunction, and describes the direction of rotation and sidebending to which it moves more freely.

► REVIEW QUESTIONS

1. Select the item that is not a component of somatic dysfunction.
   A. Characteristics of TART
   B. Congenital skeletal anomaly
   C. Neurophysiological phenomenon
   D. Responds appropriately to OMT
   E. Disturbance of the normal function of somatic structures

2. A 77-year-old male comes to see you for neck pain. You begin by observing his active and passive cervical range of motion. What is the correct association between these tests and the barrier concept?
   A. The neutral point is the point which occurs freely at the end of each motion range.
   B. The passive range of motion engages the restrictive barrier.
   C. The pathological neutral is a functional restriction at the end of a range of motion which restricts the physiological range of motion.
   D. The active range of motion engages the soft tissue restrictions of the physiological barrier.
   E. Direct techniques engage the anatomical barrier.

3. Name the terminology for the following definitions below.
   A. Two adjacent vertebrae and all of their associated components
   B. A spinal curve consisting of at least three vertebrae
   C. Describes the position of the vertebra when it is rotated and refers to the side of the prominent transverse process
   D. Describes the position of the vertebra when it is rotated and refers to the side of the less prominent transverse process
   E. The maintenance of a pool of neurons in a state of partial or subthreshold excitation

4. Please choose the incorrect statement regarding Fryette's principles.
   A. Fryette's principles describe typical spinal motion of a vertebral segment and groups of segments.
   B. Typical vertebral segments are those which have articular facets and an intervertebral disc.
   C. Fryette's Principle I applies to a neutral group where rotation and sidebending occur in opposite directions.
   D. Fryette's Principle II applies to two vertebrae in nonneutral where rotation and sidebending occur to the same side.
   E. The occiput follows the motion of Principle II.

5. If in the office you find that your patient has a flexed T3 vertebrae rotated and sidebent to the right side, which of the following statements would be incorrect about your finding?
   A. The segment is named according to its relative position to the vertebra below.
   B. You would notate your finding as T3FRSR.
   C. The most posterior inferior aspect if the vertebral body is used as the nomenclature frame of reference.
   D. T3 would move more freely in flexion.
   E. T3 would be restricted in its rotation and sidebending to the left.

▶ ANSWERS

1. **B**

Somatic dysfunction is a disturbance of somatic structures that responds to treatment by OMT. A patient with a congenital anomaly may experience a benefit in well-being by treatment with OMT, but the congenital deformity is not an example of somatic dysfunction.

2. **D**

For answer A, the neutral point is the point at which quality and quantity of motion are equal on both sides. For B, the passive range of motion engages the anatomical barrier. For C, the pathological neutral is the neutral point that exists which is present with a loss of range of motion on one side. For answer D, direct techniques engage the restrictive barrier and should never engage the anatomical barrier.

3. **A,** Vertebral unit. **B,** Group curve. **C,** Posterior component. **D,** Anterior component. **E,** Facilitation.

4. **E**

The occiput is not a typical vertebral segment. It also rotates and sidebends to opposite sides.

5. **C**

The most anterior superior aspect of the vertebral body is used as the frame of reference.

Overview of Techniques

This chapter provides a review of the major osteopathic manipulative technique modalities that have been developed. While there are many others being developed and used, only those most commonly taught have been included. Osteopathy in the cranial field is covered in its own chapter (see Chapter 4). Most of the information in this chapter is distilled from the second edition of *Foundations for Osteopathic Medicine*; however, the organization and classification differ slightly. A description of specific techniques can be found in Chapter 7. This chapter is divided into four sections:

- Overview of techniques—categories and comparisons
- Summary table of techniques
- Details of techniques
- Review questions

▶ OVERVIEW OF TECHNIQUES—CATEGORIES AND COMPARISONS

Given all of the techniques that exist, it can be confusing to sort them and keep them straight. Much of the confusion arises from the similarities that exist among many of the techniques. One helpful way of categorizing techniques is dividing them between **direct** and **indirect**. A **direct** action technique is one that engages a physiologically restricted barrier and attempts to "break through" the barrier by directly engaging it. With **indirect** technique, the body is positioned away from the barrier to allow restrictive tissues to release inherently (see Barrier Concept in Chapter 2). With the tissues released, there is no longer a restrictive barrier. Not all indirect techniques deal with barriers, however. They may also be used to release reactive tissues in the absence of joint dysfunction. Table 3-1 summarizes techniques by direct and indirect.

Below are some of the features that differentiate the techniques. As with any brief comparison, these are generalizations and not absolutes.

Direct Techniques

- High velocity, low amplitude (**HVLA**) and **articulation** are entirely passive—the physician does all the work.
- **Muscle energy (ME)** is both active and passive—the physician and patient both work.
- **HVLA** requires firm barrier engagement.
- **ME** engages initial barrier resistance—the feather edge.
- All of the techniques may use multiple planes to engage the barrier. In **ME** and **articulation**, the barriers in the three cardinal planes may be engaged either individually or in combination.

TABLE 3-1. **Technique Classifications**

DIRECT	INDIRECT	BOTH
HVLA	Strain and CS	MFR
ME	FPR	
ART	BLT	

ART, articulation; BLT, balanced ligamentous tension; CS, counterstrain; FPR, facilitated positional release; HVLA, high velocity, low amplitude; ME, muscle energy; MFR, myofascial release.

Indirect Techniques

- All techniques may address tenderness, but **counterstrain** has specific tenderpoints.
- Myofascial release (**MFR**) releases soft tissues; this may (or may not) be with the intention of freeing up a specific joint.
- Facilitated positional release (**FPR**) is very similar to **MFR**, but adds a facilitating force to expedite the process.
- Balanced ligamentous tension (**BLT**) specifically deals with balancing the ligamentous tissues of a joint.

Active motion is motion carried out by the patient. Passive motion is motion carried out by the physician.

▶ **SUMMARY OF TECHNIQUES**

Technique	Summary
HVLA	- Also known as thrust technique - Used to remove articular restriction to motion—static asymmetry alone is not a sufficient indication - Patient is positioned such that the dysfunctional joint engages the restricted barrier and a quick thrust—high velocity—over a very short distance—low amplitude—is applied by the practitioner
ME	- A direct technique in which the physician engages the initial resistance to a barrier—the feather edge—and asks the patient to provide a counterforce away from the barrier - Forces are generally light—excessive force is a common error - The active contraction by the patient acts to mobilize a joint directly or by providing a postisometric relaxation period whereby tissues can be further stretched
ART	- Gentle, repetitive, and passive motion of a joint into its restricted barrier and through its range of motion to "loosen" the joint - Examples include Spencer technique for the shoulder and rib raising
MFR	- A direct or indirect approach to releasing tension in muscles (myo) and fascia (fascial) - With a direct approach, tissue barriers are engaged rhythmically, or engaged and held - With an indirect approach, tissues are taken to a place where the least amount of tension exists and held until an inherent release occurs
Strain and CS	- Treatment consists of positioning the patient to eliminate the tenderness and tension—a position of ease—and holding this for 90 seconds - More than 200 specific points found anteriorly and posteriorly. Usually discrete, fingertip size, tense, and edematous. Patient will typically wince because of exquisite tenderness of significant points - Tenderpoints typically in tendons or muscle belly. They may also be found in other myofascial tissues - If multiple tenderpoints are found, treat the most tender point first - Points are often away from a point of trauma. For example, tenderpoints on the chest wall with back pain, or points in the antagonist muscle of a traumatized muscle - If pain is associated with trauma, position of treatment matches the position of trauma and is associated with maximal comfort

Technique	Summary
BLT	▪ An indirect approach where tensions of the ligaments and membranous structures are balanced by joint positioning. This allows an inherent release in the tissues ▪ Active movement by the patient—often breath—is commonly used to assist with the release
FPR	▪ A form of indirect treatment—positional release—in which a facilitating force is added to decrease the amount of treatment time needed ▪ Facilitating force is compression and or torsion ▪ Used for both tissue texture change and joint restriction secondary to myofascial tension ▪ Treatment always begins with putting joint into a neutral position then adding a facilitating force

ART, articulation; BLT, balanced ligamentous tension; CS, counterstrain; FPR, facilitated positional release; HVLA, high velocity, low amplitude; ME, muscle energy; MFR, myofascial release.

▶ **DETAILS OF TECHNIQUES**

High Velocity, Low Amplitude

- **Description**: A direct technique, which moves a joint through a restricted barrier with high velocity—a quick, sudden impulse, and low amplitude—the extent of movement is very small. The technique is used to remove articular restrictions to motion.
- **Indications**: Restriction of a joint to active and or passive motion testing. Static asymmetry alone is not a sufficient indication for HVLA.
- **Contraindications/Precautions**:
  - Hypermobile joints (the technique may work, but it may contribute to joint instability which accompanies hypermobility).
  - Traumatic muscle contracture.
  - Bone fracture.
  - Advanced degenerative joint disease (DJD) and or ankylosis.
  - A rubbery or indistinct barrier is usually an indication that a thrust will be ineffective.
  - A patient who is unable to relax the muscles around the joint.
  - Osteoporosis and discs are not necessarily absolute contraindications, but are indications for trying other approaches first.
- **Typical sequence**:
  1. Position patient such that the restricted joint is into the restricted barrier. It is important that the barrier is firmly engaged so there is no windup preceding the thrust.
  2. Practitioner performs a quick thrust over a short distance into the restricted barrier forcing the joint through the restriction. This may (or may not) be accompanied by a pop.
  3. Reassess for increased joint mobility and decreased TART.
- **Final activating force**: Practitioner force into the restricted barrier
- **Examples**:
  - Kirksville crunch
  - Crosshand pisiform
  - Talar tug
  - Hiss plantar whip

An indistinct or rubbery end feel may indicate muscle hypertonicity. Other techniques such as MFR, ME, or articulation may be needed to prepare the joint for HVLA. An indistinct or rubbery end feel may indicate a viscerosomatic reflex.

Muscle Energy

- **Description**: A direct technique in which a patient's active muscle force is used to affect somatic change in a desired way. This technique requires very specific positioning of the patient, and a physician counterforce to the patient's muscle force. The technique is used to:
  - Decrease joint restriction
  - Decrease muscle hypertonicity and lengthen muscle fibers
  - Reduce restrictions to respiratory inhalation/exhalation
  - Strengthen weaknesses that produce asymmetry
- Categories (amount of force to be used):
  - **Joint mobilization** (30-50 lb)—patient's muscle contraction mobilizes joint.
  - **Postisometric relaxation** (10-20 lb)—following contraction, muscles are relaxed and can be further stretched.
  - **Respiratory assistance**—exaggerated breathing as a muscle force.
  - **Oculocephalogyric reflex** (ounces)—eye movements reflexively affect muscles of neck and trunk.
  - **Reciprocal inhibition** (ounces)—agonist contraction produces reflex relaxation of the antagonist group.
  - **Crossed extensor reflex** (ounces)—contraction of flexor in an extremity produces relaxation of flexor and contraction of extensor in contralateral extremity.
- **Indications**: Asymmetry of joint motion and/or muscle hypertonicity.
- **Contraindications/Precautions**:
  - Acute injury*
  - Pain in muscle*
  - Patient too young to cooperate
  - Patient unresponsive
  - Patient cannot understand or follow instructions
- **Typical sequence**:
  1. Position body part to position of initial resistance (**feather edge**).
  2. Instruct patient to contract against the physician force.
  3. Maintain force for 3 to 5 seconds.
  4. Patient instructed to release force of contraction slowly. Physician releases force along with patient.
  5. Wait several seconds for the tissues to relax. The physician then takes up the slack into a new barrier of initial resistance.
  6. Repeat steps 2 through 5, three to five times.
  7. Reassess for increased joint motion or decreased muscle tension.
- **Final activating force**: Contraction of patient's muscles either moves a joint or provides for a postisometric relaxation period whereby tissues can be further stretched.

Feather edge is a term often applied to ME. It is defined as the point where the physician first feels restriction to motion. This restriction is caused by soft-tissue restriction and has a different end feeling than that felt with HVLA in which a distinct articular barrier is felt. Excessive force is a common error made when employing ME technique.

Articulation

- **Description**: Gentle, repetitive, and passive motion of a joint into its restricted barrier to "loosen" the joint. The goal is to reduce the resistance to motion (usually tight connective tissue), and improve or restore normal physiological motion. It may also be used simultaneously, or as a stand-alone diagnostic tool.

---

*May still be able to use reciprocal inhibition or crossed extensor reflex techniques.

- **Indications:** Restriction to articular movement. Good for postoperative or older, immobile patients when tolerated.
- **Contraindications/Precautions:**
  - Generally a safe technique
  - Pain (other than mild soreness or mild discomfort) with technique
  - Sutures, burns, infections, or other acute injury in area of treatment
  - Traumatic muscle contracture or bone fracture
  - Advanced DJD and or ankylosis—use with caution
- **Typical sequence:**
  1. With the patient in a comfortable position, the physician gently moves the joint to the restricted barrier or to the limit of the patient's tolerance.
  2. The joint is then returned to neutral and this whole process is repeated in a rhythmic pattern.
  3. With each repetition, the range of motion should increase. Once there is no further increase in motion, the treatment is finished.
- **Final activating force:** Direct and repetitive stretching of restrictive tissues by the physician
- **Examples:**
  - Rib raising
  - Spencer technique for the shoulder
  - Thoracic lymphatic pump

Very young and very old respond well to articulation. Usually less posttreatment reaction than with HVLA.

Myofascial Release

- **Description:** Strictly speaking, it is the release of tension in muscles (myo) and fascia (fascial). This is achieved by applying a direct force to stretch tissues or an indirect force to allow an inherent release of the tissues. Also included in this category is **inhibition** that works by maintaining deep pressure over an area of hypertonicity.
- **Indications:** Muscular and or fascial restrictions. This may include joint restrictions, which are caused by or held by hypertonic tissues. It can be used to "prepare" a joint for HVLA or as a stand-alone technique.
- **Contraindications/Precautions:**
  - Generally a safe technique
  - Pain (other than mild soreness or mild discomfort) with technique
  - Sutures, burns, infections, or other acute injury in area of treatment
- **Typical sequence:**
  - **Direct**
    1. Engage tissues with pressure appropriate to depth of interest.
    2. Move them into a restricted barrier and hold the stretch or allow tissues to relax and repeat stretching in a rhythmic manner. The barrier may be engaged with any of the following motions: translation, rotation, distraction, compression.
  - **Indirect**
    1. Engage tissues with pressure appropriate to depth of interest.
    2. Move tissues to a point of least resistance. This may include any of the following: translation, rotation, distraction, compression.
    3. Wait for an inherent release in the tissues.
- **Final activating force:**
  - Direct—stretching from the force of physician's manipulation
  - Indirect—an inherent release of the patient's tissues

In order to maximize the release, direct and indirect approaches are often used together in a combined approach (start indirect and go direct).

Strain and Counterstrain

(See also Chapter 6 for Jones' Counterstrain Tenderpoints.)

- **Description:** The use of gentle positioning to maximally decrease tenderness of specific tenderpoints in order to restore normal somatic function. There are more than 200 discrete but specific anatomical points, anteriorly and posteriorly, which can be found in muscles, tendons, and ligaments.
- **Indications:** Presence of a tenderpoint.
- **Contraindications/Precautions:**
  - Generally a safe technique
  - Pain (other than mild soreness or mild discomfort) with technique
  - Sutures, burns, infections, or other acute injury in area of treatment
- **Typical sequence:**
  1. Slowly move patient to position of comfort while monitoring for tissue relaxation. Monitoring should be done with a light touch.
  2. Determine degree of tenderness by pressing the tenderpoint and asking patient for the level of tenderness still present. **On a 0 to 10 scale, tenderness should reduce from an initial value of 10, to a 3 or less. If greater than a 3, fine-tune until tenderness decreases.** *
  3. Maintain position for 90 seconds and monitor tissues for a sensation of release.
  4. Following **90 seconds** and/or release, slowly return patient to neutral. It is important that the patient remains passive during this return.
  5. Recheck tenderpoint for tenderness. **A successful treatment leaves no more than 30% of the original tenderness.**
- **Final activating force:** An inherent release of the patient's tissues.

Light contact throughout treatment sequence should be maintained. Pressure is used only to determine the degree of tenderness. Midline points generally require more flexion/extension. Lateral points generally require more sidebending/rotation.

Balanced Ligamentous Tension

- **Description:** Indirect positioning of a dysfunctional joint to a place of balanced ligamentous and membranous tensions. In practice this means that when a balance point is achieved, any additional motion will create an imbalance of tension around the joint. Finding this point of balance will allow inherent forces to correct the dysfunction and the tissues will return to a physiologically correct balance point. Active movement from the patient (especially breath) is often used to achieve this balance and help with the release.
- **Indications:** Restriction or asymmetry of motion in any articulation.
- **Contraindications/Precautions:**
  - Generally a safe technique
  - Pain (other than mild soreness or mild discomfort) with technique
  - Sutures, burns, infections, or other acute injury in area of treatment
- **Typical sequence:**
  1. After finding a restriction in movement of a joint, the patient's body is positioned to find a point of balance in the ligamentous tensions.
     - This may include active motion by the patient to tune the balance. As the patient returns to neutral, the joint is held in position by the physician until a release occurs.

Notes for BLT:

- Respiratory assistance
- Inhalation flattens the spine in the AP direction (ie, thoracic kyphosis and lumbar lordosis decrease).
- Exhalation increases AP spinal curves.
- In this model, ligaments of a joint neither stretch nor go lax as long as the joint stays within physiological limits.
- The degree of motion required is very small for diagnosis and treatment.
- First described by W.G. Sutherland, DO, in the 1940s.

---

* If fine-tuning is not working, one can treat the paired point (ie, if you are treating an anterior point without success, treat its corresponding posterior point) and then return to treating the original point.

  - Alternatively, breathing may be used to tune the balance. For example, an inhale flattens spinal curves (in anteroposterior [AP] direction) and can be used to extend upper thoracics (above T8) or flex lower thoracics. Once balance is achieved, the balance point is held for several respiratory cycles until it self-corrects.
    2. Correction of the dysfunction is sensed when the point of balance shifts back toward the normal physiological neutral.
    3. Reassess joint movement and symmetry.
  - **Final activating force**: Inherent physiological forces. Often this is breathing.

Facilitated Positional Release

- **Description**: A specific form of indirect treatment in which a facilitating force (usually compression or torsion) is used to reduce the time needed for the tissues to release. It can be used to resolve tissue texture changes as well as joint dysfunction resulting from muscle hypertonicity.
- **Indications**: Tissue texture change and joint dysfunction secondary to tissue hypertonicity.
- **Contraindications/Precautions**:
  - Generally a safe technique
  - Pain (other than mild soreness or mild discomfort) with technique
  - Sutures, burns, infections, or other acute injury in area of treatment
- Typical sequence:
  1. The dysfunctional joint is placed into a neutral position to unload articular surfaces. For vertebra, neutral relates to a position between flexed and extended.
  2. A facilitating force (compression and or torsion) is applied.
  3. The tissues are further placed in a position of relative freedom to allow them to "relax."
  4. In a matter of several seconds, the dysfunction resolves and the joint can be returned to the original position.
  5. Reassess for resolution of dysfunction.
- **Final activating force**: An inherent release of the patient's tissues.

▶ REVIEW QUESTIONS

Name the technique associated with each of the following descriptions.

A. Compression or torsion added to expedite the release
B. Articular barrier firmly engaged
C. Hold for 90 seconds
D. Active movement by patient (often breath) to find a balance point
E. Feather edge of a barrier engaged

▶ ANSWERS

A, FPR. B, HVLA or articulation. C, Counterstrain. D, BLT. E, Muscle energy.

Regional and Systems-Based Assessment

▶ Regional Diagnosis

▶ Osteopathic Principles
and Considerations of
Clinical Medicine:
A Systems-Based
Approach

CHAPTER 4

Regional Diagnosis

Osteopathic manipulative medicine (OMM) questions in the Comprehensive Osteopathic Medical Licensing Examination (COMLEX) often reveal findings of a structural examination or present different restrictions in the various regions of the body. It is your job to determine what the true diagnosis is. This section will review the principles and guidelines for diagnosing somatic dysfunctions (SDs) and other structural abnormalities throughout the body.

Primary respiratory mechanism (PRM) was first described by William G. Sutherland, DO.

- Primary = vegetative center of the brain
- Respiratory = metabolic exchange at the cellular level
- Mechanism = an integrated machine

The five components of PRM are

- Inherent motility of the brain is considered to be the driving force.
- Cerebrospinal fluid (CSF) is the hydraulic aspect, moving in a concurrent fashion.
- Articular motility of the bones of the skull.
- Mobility of the membranes and the reciprocal tension membrane (RTM).
- Involuntary motion of the sacrum.

Relevant Anatomy

(See Figures 4-1, 4-2, 4-3, 4-4.)

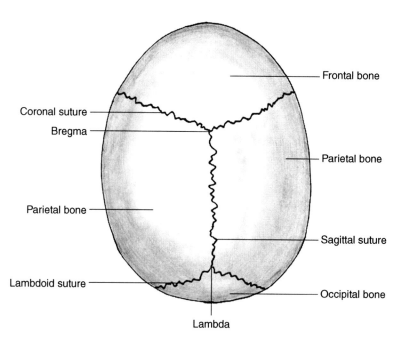

Coronal suture
Bregma
Parietal bone
Lambdoid suture
Lambda
Frontal bone
Parietal bone
Sagittal suture
Occipital bone

FIGURE 4-1. Cranium—superior view.

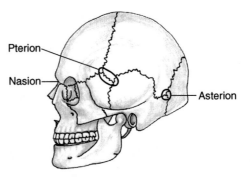

FIGURE 4-2. **Cranium—lateral view.**

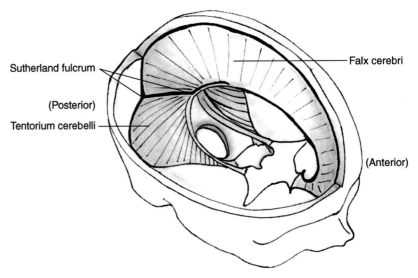

FIGURE 4-3. **The dural septa.**

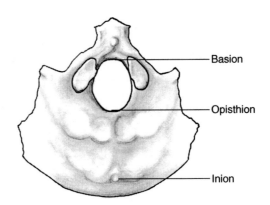

FIGURE 4-4. **Occiput.**

BONY

Midline bones = sphenoid, occiput, sacrum
Paired bones = frontal, parietal, temporal, nasal, zygoma, maxilla

CONNECTIVE TISSUE

- Falx cerebri, tentorium cerebelli, and spinal dura form RTM.
- Falx cerebri and tentorium cerebelli arise from a common origin at the straight sinus known as the Sutherland fulcrum. This point is not actually a detectable structure. An analogy would be the "center of gravity" in the body.
- Dura continues down the spinal canal and attaches to the sacrum at the level of S2.
- The RTM attaches anteriorly at the cribriform plate and crista galli of the ethmoid bone, as well as the clinoid processes of the sphenoid, posteriorly at the occiput, and laterally at the petrous portion of the temporal bones.

LANDMARKS

- Sphenobasilar synchondrosis (SBS): Junction of body of sphenoid and body of occiput; point about which flexion and extension occurs
- Pterion: Junction of frontal, sphenoid, parietal, and temporal bones
- Asterion: Junction of occiput, parietal, temporal bones
- Basion: Ventral aspect of foramen magnum
- Opisthion: Dorsal aspect of foramen magnum
- Inion: Occipital protuberance
- Nasion: Junction of nasal and frontal bones
- Bregma: Junction of coronal and sagittal sutures

CRANIAL MOTION

- Primary movements of SBS are flexion and extension.
- During flexion, SBS rises; during extension, SBS falls (Figure 4-5).
- In flexion, the body of the sphenoid rises and moves slightly anterior. The wings move anterior and laterally, while moving slightly inferior.
- In flexion, the base of the occiput rises and moves slightly posterior. The squamous portion of the occiput moves inferior and laterally.
- Sphenoid and occiput circumduct in opposite directions about two transverse axes (Figure 4-5).

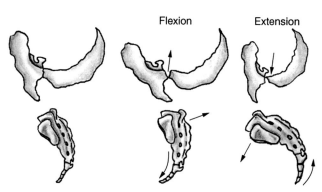

Flexion   Extension

FIGURE 4-5.   **Cranial flexion and extension of the SBS and sacrum.**

*Occipital landmarks **BOIL** Basion, Opisthion, Inion, Lambdoidal suture.*

- Paired bones externally rotate (lateral aspect of bones move away from the midline) in flexion and internally rotate (lateral aspect of bones move toward the midline) in extension.
- Occiput influences motion and direction of temporals, mandible, and sacrum.
- Sphenoid influences motion and direction of anterior cranium including frontals, ethmoid, maxilla, zygoma, vomer, and palatine bone.

SACRAL MOTION

- Sacrum = midline bone. It moves on a transverse axis located at the level of S2 (in the area where the lamina might be if the sacrum had lamina).
- In flexion, the sacral base moves posteriorly and superiorly.
- In extension, the sacral base moves anteriorly and inferiorly.
- The base of the sacrum and base of the occiput move in the same direction (Figure 4-5).

SPECIFIC BONE DYSFUNCTION

- Frontal bone dysfunction may often cause sinus congestion.
- Temporal bone dysfunction may cause tinnitus, vertigo, otitis, and migraine.
- Nine pairs of cranial nerves (CNs) are potentially influenced by temporal bone motion (CN III-XI).
- Compression of condylar components in a newborn may cause feeding difficulties caused by compression of CN XII.

*Mnemonic for cranial strain patterns: **T**ight **S**kull **B**ones **R**eally **L**ike **V**-Spread techniques.*

Cranial Strain Patterns

(See Table 4-1.)

- Types of strain patterns are **T**orsion, **S**idebending **R**otation, **L**ateral, **V**ertical, SBS compression.
- Strains can be palpated with either vault or anteroposterior (AP) contact.
- Two types of strain patterns: Physiological and nonphysiological.

When palpating strain patterns, do you note "healthy" flexion and extension? If yes, the strain pattern is probably physiological. If no, strain pattern is probably nonphysiological.

SPHENOBASILAR TORSION STRAIN PATTERN

(See Figure 4-6.)

- Physiological strain pattern.
- Results in rotation of the sphenoid and occiput in opposite directions about a relative AP axis.
- Named for the "high" greater wing of the sphenoid.
- While palpating a right torsion using vault contact, you will notice your right index finger is more superior (closer toward you) than your left. Your left fifth digit will be more superior (closer toward you) than your right.
- In the AP hold, you will appreciate a twisting in the falx such that one hand rotates in one direction and the other hand rotates in the opposite direction.
- Torsion = twisting of dural membranes.

TABLE 4-1. Strain Patterns

PATTERN	TORSION	SBR	LATERAL	VERTICAL	SBS COMPRESSION
Physiological/ Nonphysiological	Physiological	Physiological	Nonphysiological	Nonphysiological	Nonphysiological
Sphenoid and occiput motion	Opposite directions about AP axis	Rotate same direction about AP axis, opposite directions about two transverse axes	Same direction about two vertical axes	Same direction about two transverse axes	Severely restricted motion
Named for	High greater wing of sphenoid (right or left)	Which side is convex and inferior (down and out), (full side of head), (right or left)	Base of sphenoid in relation to base of occiput (right or left)	Base of sphenoid in relation to base of occiput (superior or inferior)	Lack of motion
What you palpate using vault contact	R-torsion = R 1st and L 5th digits move freely superiorly. L 1st and R 5th digits move freely inferiorly. Twisted falx	R SBR = R 1st and 5th digits spread and move inferior, (fullness) L 1st and 5th digits move closer and superior	R Lateral = sphenoid translates freely R, base of sphenoid carried right in relation in occiput	Superior = sphenoid in flexion, occiput in extension. Greater wings move anteriorly and inferiorly. Inferior = sphenoid in extension, occiput in flexion. Greater wings move superiorly and posteriorly	Limited motion, decreased amplitude and rate of CRI

AP, anteroposterior; CRI, cranial rhythmic impulse; L, left; R, right; SBR, sidebending rotation; SBS, sphenobasilar synchondrosis.

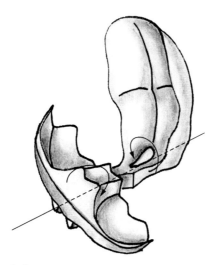

FIGURE 4-6. Torsion strain pattern.

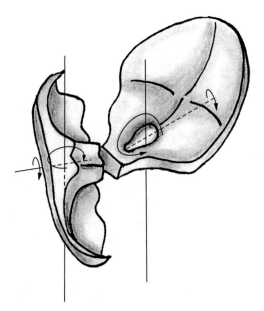

FIGURE 4-7. SBR strain pattern.

SIDEBENDING-ROTATION STRAIN PATTERNS

(See Figure 4-7.)

- Physiological strain pattern.
- Involve two main motions.
  - Motion 1: Sphenoid and occiput rotate in same direction about one AP axis.
  - Motion 2: Sphenoid and occiput sidebend away from each other, such that the "low" side forms a convexity and the "high" side forms a concavity.
- Using vault contact to palpate a right sidebending-rotation (SBR), the operator will note the fingers on the right hand separating from each other, while sensing a convexity or fullness on the right side. The left fingers will approximate and the left side of the head may feel "flat."
- Named for whichever side is low (down) and convex (out).

LATERAL STRAIN PATTERNS

(See Figure 4-8.)

- Nonphysiological (traumatic) strain pattern.
- Result when a force (eg, a blow to the temples) causes a translatory motion of the body of the sphenoid in relation to the body of the occiput.
- Cause rotation of the sphenoid and occiput in the same direction on two vertical axes, after this translatory motion has occurred.
- Named for the relationship of the base of the sphenoid in relation to the base of the occiput.

Example: Your attending becomes upset and throws a chart at you, which hits you square in your left temple. The base of your sphenoid will be displaced to the right. When you have a fellow student work on your head later, they will appreciate the sphenoid being "carried" to right relative to the position of the occiput. This would be diagnosed as a right lateral strain.

- This pattern may give a palpatory impression of a "parallelogram" head. In addition, these strains may result in the appearance of a parallelogram-shaped head in the newborn (Figure 4-9).

SBR strain patterns are named for whichever side is "down and out."

The greater wings of the sphenoid may rotate in slightly different directions depending on the vector of the force causing the lateral strain. However, on board questions, just worry about the base of the sphenoid in relation to the base of the occiput.

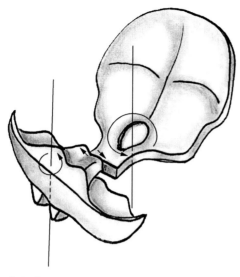

FIGURE 4-8. Lateral strain pattern.

- May be difficult to detect flexion and extension of the cranial rhythmic impulse (CRI).

VERTICAL STRAIN PATTERNS

(See Figures 4-10 and 4-11.)

- Nonphysiological (traumatic) strain patterns
- Result when a force causes a vertical (superior or inferior) displacement of the base of the sphenoid relative to the base of the occiput
- Cause rotation of the sphenoid and occiput in the same direction about two transverse axes
- Named for position of the base of the sphenoid in relation to the base of the occiput

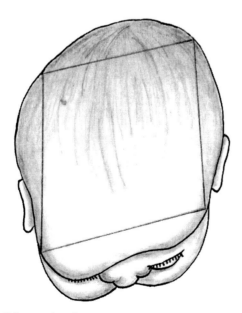

FIGURE 4-9. Parallelogram head.

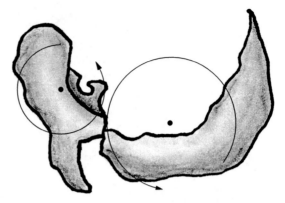

FIGURE 4-10. Superior vertical strain pattern.

SUPERIOR VERTICAL STRAIN

(See Figure 4-10.)

▪ Base of the sphenoid is superior to the base of the occiput (eg, falling on the back of your head driving your occiput anterior and inferior).
▪ While palpating the patient using vault contact, the wings of the sphenoid will move forward and lateral, as if the sphenoid was in flexion, while the occiput is in extension.

INFERIOR VERTICAL STRAIN

(See Figure 4-11.)

▪ Base of the sphenoid is inferior to the base of the occiput (eg, from standing up and hitting an open cupboard door after treating a patient in a tiny examination room).
▪ While palpating the patient using vault contact, the wings of the sphenoid will move superiorly and medial, as if the sphenoid was in extension, while the occiput is in flexion.

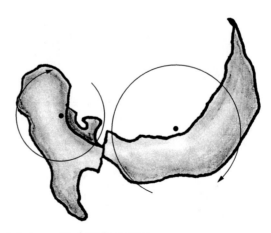

FIGURE 4-11. Inferior vertical strain pattern.

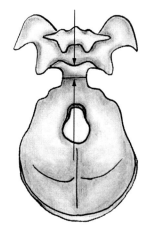

FIGURE 4-12. SBS compression.

SBS COMPRESSION

(See Figure 4-12.)

- Nonphysiological (traumatic) strain pattern.
- Results from the base of the sphenoid becoming compressed into the base of the occiput as a result of birth (ie, face presentation), trauma (ie, head on windshield), or sacral dysfunction (ie, falling on sacrum).
- Flexion and extension are limited.
- Rate and amplitude will be decreased.
- On palpation using vault or AP contact, the operator will note extremely restricted motion of the SBS. The operator may note no motion at all, suggesting a "bowling ball head."
- Can be common in newborns because of compression of the head through the birth canal.
- CV4 may be useful treatment for this strain pattern.

Table 4-1 provides a summary of the various strain patterns.

Techniques

The following techniques are discussed in detail in Chapter 7.

Vault contact
Anteroposterior contact
Sacral contact
V-spread
CV4 technique
Frontal lift

Name vertical strains for the base of the sphenoid in relation to the base of the occiput, not the wings.

► REVIEW QUESTIONS: CRANIAL DIAGNOSIS

Questions 1–2

A 33-year-old patient comes to see you for osteopathic manipulative techniques (OMT). During your treatment, the patient tells you he has been feeling generally tired and fatigued recently. He has no previous trauma history except a recent fall on the ice but he didn't hit his head. You check his cranial motion and note a dramatic decrease in amplitude and rate of the CRI.

1. Which bone(s) involved in cranial motion may be responsible for these findings?
   A. Occiput
   B. Temporal bones
   C. Parietal bones
   D. Frontal bones
   E. Sacrum

2. What may be an appropriate treatment for this strain pattern?
   A. Frontal lift
   B. CV4
   C. V-spread
   D. Temporal balancing
   E. No treatment is necessary

Questions 3–4

A 28-year-old patient comes to see you after a several-year history of indigestion, gas, and intermittent diarrhea. In addition to a thorough workup, you decide to examine the patient's cranial motion.

3. You are concerned that the _____ may be compressing CN _____.
   A. Jugular foramen, IX
   B. Jugular foramen, X
   C. Jugular foramen, XI
   D. Stylomastoid foramen, VII
   E. Stylomastoid foramen, VIII

4. During normal flexion and extension, the occiput and sphenoid usually
   A. Rotate in the same direction about two transverse axes
   B. Rotate in the same direction about two vertical axes
   C. Rotate in the same direction about one AP axis
   D. Rotate in opposite directions about two vertical axes
   E. Rotate in opposite directions about two transverse axes

5. A patient comes to see you after having a cold for several days. During your examination, she mentions she has been very dizzy and has had ringing in her ears lately. What might you expect to find on cranial palpation?
   A. CRI rate of 26/min
   B. Internally rotated temporal bone
   C. Flexed parietal bone
   D. Externally rotated ethmoid bone
   E. Internally rotated sacrum

6. In motion testing your patient's head, you note the following findings: Your left index finger and pinky come together and move toward you, while your right index finger and pinky spread apart and move away from you. What strain pattern are you palpating?
   A. SBS compression
   B. Right torsion strain
   C. Right SBR strain
   D. Superior vertical strain
   E. Right lateral strain

7. A patient comes to see you after complaining of headaches. While palpating the patient's cranium, you notice your left pinky and right index finger move superiorly. Which is true regarding this strain pattern?
   A. It involves rotation in opposite directions about two superior axes.
   B. It involves rotation in opposite directions about an AP axis.
   C. It is nonphysiological (traumatic).
   D. It is named for the relationship of the base of the sphenoid in relationship to the base of the occiput.
   E. It often results from a blow to the top of the head or under the chin.

8. Your classmate finds you at the hospital you both are rotating at after a demented patient gave him an uppercut to the chin. While palpating, you note both wings of the sphenoid move freely inferiorly. Which statement is true regarding this strain pattern?
   A. It is named for the free motion of the wings of the sphenoid.
   B. The occiput and sphenoid rotate in the same direction about an AP axis.
   C. This is a physiological strain.
   D. As the sphenoid flexes, the sacral base moves posterior.
   E. The occiput moves in the same direction as the sphenoid about two transverse axes.

▶ ANSWERS

1. **E**

Judging from the history and the presentation, a locked sacrum is most likely at the root of this patient's compression.

2. **B**

CV4 is a useful technique for increasing the overall rate and amplitude of the CRI.

3. **B**

The jugular foramen houses many structures, including CN IX, X, and XI. Judging from this person's complaints, the vagus nerve appears to be involved.

4. **E**

During flexion and extension, the sphenoid and occiput rotate in opposite directions about two transverse axes. If rotation about the AP or superior axis occurs, there is usually a strain pattern present. In vertical strain patterns, the sphenoid and occiput rotate in the same direction about two transverse axes.

5. **B**

Whenever you see tinnitus on a question involving cranial diagnosis, the first bone that comes to mind should be the temporal bone.

6. **C**

This type of question is very common on boards. The question gives you information about what you are feeling using vault contact, and how you must determine the strain pattern. Given the description of your fingers spreading and moving away from you on one side and approximating and moving toward you on the other, this sounds like a SBR strain pattern.

7. **B**

This is a two-step question. First, you must determine the strain pattern based on the information given. Second, you must remember the motion and axes involved in this strain pattern. The description of one index finger and one pinky both moving superiorly should make you think of torsion. Then, you must remember that torsion involves the sphenoid and occiput rotating in opposite directions about a relative AP axis. Choice A describes a SBR pattern. We know torsion is a physiological strain pattern, so we can rule out choice C. Choice D describes lateral and vertical strain patterns. Choice E describes vertical strain patterns.

8. **E**

This is another two-step question. We know from the history and physical examination that this is a superior vertical strain. Choice E is the only answer that fits this strain pattern. Choice A is incorrect, as these patterns are named for the base of the sphenoid. Choice B describes a SBR strain pattern. We know a vertical strain is a nonphysiological strain pattern so we can rule out choice C. Choice D is incorrect because the sacrum follows the occiput, and we know that a superior vertical strain involves a flexed sphenoid with an extended occiput. Therefore, as the sphenoid flexes, the occiput extends. As the occiput extends, the sacral base moves anterior.

▶ CERVICAL DIAGNOSIS

Relevant Anatomy

BONY

OCCIPUT

(See Figure 4-4.)

- Occipital condyles are convex and converge anteriorly.
- Condyles glide anteriorly and posteriorly in the superior articulations of the atlas causing flexion and extension of the joint.

ATLAS

(See Figure 4-13.)

- Atypical cervical segment that lacks a body and spinous process.
- Superior articulations are concave to receive occipital condyles.

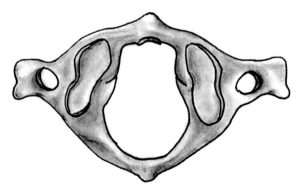

FIGURE 4-13. Atlas.

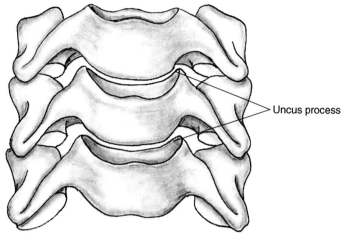

Uncus process

FIGURE 4-14. C2 to C7.

C2 TO C7

(See Figure 4-14.)

- Bodies contain uncinate processes; bodies appear concave in the coronal plane.
- Vertebral artery travels through transverse foramina.

MUSCULAR

POSTERIOR

Trapezius

- Originates on the occipital bone and all cervical and thoracic spinous processes
- Inserts on the clavicle and scapula

Levator Scapulae

- Originates on the transverse process of upper cervical vertebrae
- Inserts on superior, medial aspect of scapula

Splenius

- Originates from upper thoracic and lower cervical spinous processes
- Inserts on upper cervical transverse processes and the mastoid process of the skull
- Extends, rotates, and sidebends to the same side

Deep Muscles of the Neck (ie, erector spinae, semispinalis, and multifidus)

- Have slips that run from the thoracic spine and rib angles to the cervical spine, occiput, and mastoid process
- Mainly extend, but also rotate and sidebend the cervical spine

Suboccipital Muscles

- Rectus capitus posterior major and minor
- Obliquus capitus superior and inferior
- Extend and rotate occipito-atlantal (OA) and atlanto-axial joints

ANTERIOR

Sternocleidomastoid

- Originates on the sternum and clavicle
- Inserts on the mastoid process of the skull
- Flexes, sidebends, and rotates the head in opposite directions

Scalenes

- Anterior, middle, and posterior
- Originate on transverse processes of cervical vertebrae
- Insert on first (anterior and middle) and second (posterior) ribs
- Flex and sidebend the neck
- Brachial plexus and subclavian artery pass between anterior and middle scalenes

The majority of the muscular anatomy in the neck has extensive thoracic as well as cervical attachments. Therefore, clinical treatment of the neck typically involves both the cervical and thoracic spine.

Prevertebral Muscles

- Longus capitis, longus coli, rectus capitus anterior, and lateralis
- Main action is flexion of the neck
- May become strained in whiplash injury

FASCIA

- Superficial cervical fascia: Lymphatics must penetrate this fascia.
- Deep cervical fascia = investing, prevertebral, pretracheal.
- Pretracheal fascia is continuous with the carotid sheaths. Prevertebral fascia is continuous with the axillary sheaths (which surround the brachial plexus).

Treatment of this fascia is important in maintaining appropriate neurovascular flow of the neck.

NERVOUS

- There are eight cervical nerves.
- Nerves exit above the vertebrae; the eighth nerve exits below C7.

Active Range of Motion

- Flexion: 90°
- Extension: 70°
- Sidebending: 35° to 45°
- Rotation: 90°

Diagnosis

The cervical spine contains three major anatomical areas that each possesses different motion characteristics. Each area involves atypical Fryette mechanics, as traditional Type I and Type II motion are not found in the cervical spine.

Occiput on Atlas (C1)

(See Figure 4-15.)
 This joint does not follow Type I Fryette's principles as it rotates and sidebends in opposite directions, whether in neutral, flexion, or extension.

- Major motion is flexion/extension.
- Fifty percent of cervical flexion occurs at this joint.
- Minor motion is sidebending and rotation.

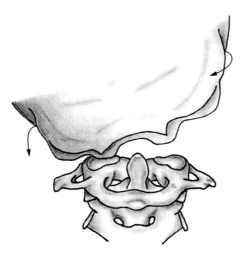

FIGURE 4-15. Occiput on atlas (C1) joint motion: rotated right, sidebent left.

Diagnosis of the occiput on the atlas can be obtained using a simple set of steps.

- Step one: Motion test the occiput.
  - This step lets you know how the occiput is moving as a whole, which helps narrow down your diagnosis.
  - Questions will typically give you some information about the motion of the occiput. Since you know the occiput rotates and sidebends in opposite directions, knowing one of these motions allows you to determine the other.
- Step two: Determine the area of greatest tissue texture change.
  - Once you know the overall motion of the occiput, determining the side of greatest tissue texture change helps determine which side of the occiput is dysfunctional.

Example: If the occiput is rotated right, sidebent left, the dysfunction will either be a posterior (flexed) occiput on the right, or an anterior (extended) occiput on the left (one of these must be occurring to cause the occiput to rotate right and sidebend left).

- To help visualize this concept, think of a patient's head sidebent left and rotated right. The right part of the occiput is closer to the treatment table (posterior), while the left side of the occiput is closer to the ceiling (anterior). For boards, those are the only two diagnostic possibilities if the occiput is sidebent left and rotated right. The opposite would be true if the occiput is sidebent right and rotated left (ie, left posterior or right anterior).
- If the tissue texture change is greatest on the right, we most likely have a posterior right occiput.
- If the tissue texture change is greatest on the left, we most likely have an anterior left occiput.
- Step three: Motion test each condyle individually.
  - Determining the motion of each condyle helps confirm which side of the occiput is dysfunctional. In addition, if no information about tissue texture change is given, this may be the only way to determine the dysfunctional condyle.

■ Again, if we assume the occiput is rotated right and sidebent left, we will either have a posterior (flexed) occiput on the right or an anterior (extended) occiput on the left.
■ If the right condyle moves freely in flexion and extension, but the left condyle is restricted in flexion, we know we have an anterior (extended) occiput on the left.
■ If the left condyle moves freely in flexion and extension, but the right condyle is restricted in extension, we know we have a posterior (flexed) occiput on the right.

EXAMPLE 1

■ The occiput is freer in left sidebending. This tells you the occiput is sidebent left and rotated right (the occiput always rotates and sidebends in opposite directions). This narrows the possible dysfunctions to two possibilities: posterior (flexed) right occiput or anterior (extended) left occiput (Figure 4-15).
■ There is increased tissue texture change and tenderness on the right. This tells us the dysfunction is on the right, and since the only possible dysfunction we can have on the right given the motion of the occiput is posterior (flexed), we know we have a posterior (flexed) occiput on the right.
■ The left condyle moves freely in flexion and extension. The right condyle moves freely in flexion but resists extension. This confirms our diagnosis of a posterior (flexed) right occiput.

EXAMPLE 2

■ The occiput is freer in left rotation. This tells you the occiput is sidebent right and rotated left. This narrows the possible dysfunctions to two possibilities: posterior (flexed) left occiput or anterior (extended) right occiput.
■ There is increased tissue texture change on the right. This tells us the dysfunction is on the right, and since the only possible dysfunction we can have on the right given the motion of the occiput is anterior (extended), we know we have an anterior (extended) occiput on the right.
■ The left condyle moves freely in both directions. The right condyle moves freely in extension but resists flexion. This confirms our diagnosis of an anterior (extended) occiput.

TREATMENT TECHNIQUES

(See Chapter 9.)

■ High velocity, low amplitude (HVLA): Occiput posterior (flexed)
■ Muscle energy (ME): Occiput posterior (flexed)
■ Indirect: Occiput posterior (flexed)

ATLAS (C1) ON AXIS (C2)

(See Figure 4-16.)

This joint does not have typical Fryette's mechanics, as the majority of motion that occurs at this joint is rotation; very little sidebending occurs here.

■ Major motion is rotation.
■ Fifty percent of cervical rotation occurs at this joint.
■ Minor motion is flexion and extension.

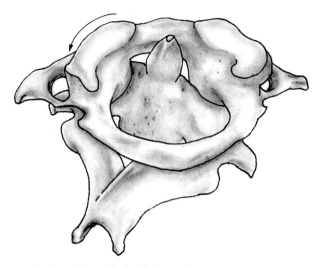

FIGURE 4-16. Atlas (C1) on axis (C2) joint motion: rotated left.

DIAGNOSIS

- Since the primary motion at the atlas is rotation, diagnosis of the atlas involves flexion of the neck to "lock out" C2 to C7, thus isolating the rotation of the neck to the atlas.
- The patient's head is rotated to the left and to the right. Freedom of motion is noted.
- If rotation to the right is greater than rotation to the left, the atlas is rotated to the right.

TREATMENT TECHNIQUES

- High velocity, low amplitude: Posterior atlas
- Muscle energy: Posterior atlas
- Indirect: Posterior atlas
- Facilitated positional release (FPR): Posterior atlas

C2 to C7

(See Figure 4-17.)

- Rotation and sidebending occur to the same side regardless of whether the spine is in neutral, flexion, or extension.

DIAGNOSIS

- Diagnosis of this region is determined by assessing motion in all three planes (ie, flexion/extension, sidebending, and rotation).

TREATMENT TECHNIQUES

- High velocity, low amplitude: Dysfunction C4FRS$_R$
- Muscle energy: Dysfunction C4FRSR$_R$
- Indirect: Dysfunction C4FRS$_R$
- Facilitated positional release: Dysfunction C4FRS$_R$

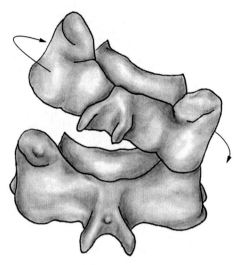

FIGURE 4-17. C3 on C4 joint motion: rotated right, sidebent right.

► **REVIEW QUESTIONS: CERVICAL DIAGNOSIS**

Questions 1–3

A 22-year-old female presents to the clinic with a complaint of headaches. After a negative workup, you diagnose her with tension headaches and decide to use OMT as an adjunctive treatment.

1. While diagnosing her occiput, you notice it sidebends freely to the right. Both condyles move freely in flexion. You diagnose
   A. Right posterior (flexed) occiput
   B. Left posterior (flexed) occiput
   C. Right anterior (extended) occiput
   D. Left anterior (extended) occiput
   E. None of the above

2. What percentage of cervical flexion occurs at the OA joint?
   A. 10%
   B. 25%
   C. 50%
   D. 75%
   E. 100%

3. The major motion of the atlas is
   A. Flexion
   B. Extension
   C. Sidebending
   D. Rotation
   E. Nutation

Questions 4–5

A 45-year-old male presents to the clinic with a history of migraines. After a negative workup, you decide to treat him using a combination of medication and OMT.

4. While palpating his occiput, you notice it rotates freely to the right. There is increased tissue texture change and tenderness over the left condyle. You diagnose
   A. Right posterior (flexed) occiput
   B. Left posterior (flexed) occiput
   C. Right anterior (extended) occiput
   D. Left anterior (extended) occiput
   E. None of the above

5. C2 to C7 rotate and sidebend to the same side in which position(s).
   A. Flexion
   B. Extension
   C. Neutral
   D. All of the above
   E. None of the above

1. **B**

This question gives us little information, but enough to make the correct diagnosis. The occiput is sidebent to the right; therefore, it is rotated to the left. This gives us two choices, B and C. Since both condyles move freely in flexion, we can rule out choice C. An anterior occiput on the right would be restricted in flexion on the right, but free in extension. A left posterior occiput is free in flexion, but resists extension on the left.

2. **C**

Fifty percent of cervical flexion occurs at the OA joint.

3. **D**

The major motion of the atlas is rotation. The minor motions of the atlas are flexion and extension. Very little sidebending occurs at the atlas. *Nutation* refers to the forward nodding of the sacrum during craniosacral extension.

4. **D**

Again, the question is not exactly forthcoming; however, we have what we need to answer it correctly. If the occiput rotates to the right, it sidebends to the left. This narrows the choices down to A and D. If we have tissue texture changes over the left aspect of the occiput, we can rule out a right-sided problem, leaving us with our answer. (Note: In reality, one cannot rule out a right-sided problem based on tissue texture changes alone. However, board questions tend to be straightforward in this manner.)

5. **D**

C2 to C7 rotate and sidebend to the same side in flexion, extension, and neutral positions.

► THORACIC, RIB, AND DIAPHRAGM DIAGNOSIS

The thoracic region is integral to most SDs. Problems in the upper thoracics can create or maintain dysfunction in the head, neck, and upper extremities. Problems in the lower thoracics can contribute to low back pain and even lower extremity complaints. Breathing and thus many lymphatic issues are centered here. Finally, given that sympathetic dorsal root ganglion are primarily located in the thoracic spine, viscerosomatic reflexes are an important consideration in this location. (See Chapter 6 for a review of viscerosomatic reflexes.)

Landmarks

POSTERIOR

- C7: Vertebra prominens
- T3: Spine of scapula
- T7: Inferior angle of scapula

ANTERIOR

- Sternal notch at level of T2
- Sternal angle at level of T4
- Xyphoid process at level of T9

Rule of 3s

(See Figure 4-18.)

- **T1 to T3**: Spinous processes lie at level of same vertebral body
- **T4 to T6**: Spinous processes lie at level between associated vertebral body and one segment below

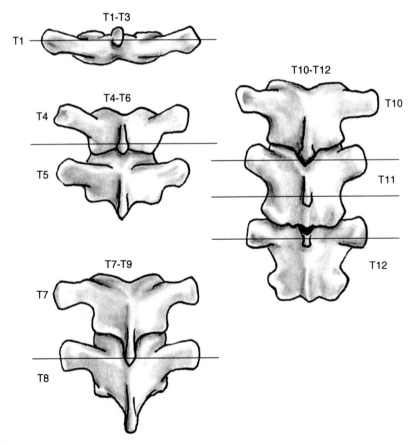

FIGURE 4-18. **Rule of 3s.**

- **T7 to T9**: Spinous processes lie at level of the vertebral body one segment below
- **T10**: Same as T7 to T9, **T11**:Same as T4 to T6, **T12**: Same as T1 to T3

Diagnosis and Treatment

This section will be divided into three areas:

1. Thoracic spine
2. Ribs
3. Diaphragm

THORACIC SPINE

RELEVANT ANATOMY

Bony

Twelve vertebrae

- All vertebral segments have the same basic architecture, which consists of a body, pedicles, laminae, transverse processes, superior and inferior facets, and a spinous process (Figure 4-19).
- The orientations of the facet joints remain constant. The inferior articular facet of the vertebra above lies over the superior articular facet of the vertebra below (as viewed from behind) in the same way that roof shingles lie.

ACTIVE RANGE OF MOTION

- Flexion: 20° to 45°
- Extension: 25° to 45°
- Sidebending: 20° to 40°
- Rotation: 35° to 50°

DIAGNOSIS

- When diagnosing the thoracic spine, any of the following may be observed:
- Anteroposterior curves—**kyphosis**
  - An increased kyphosis is generally the result of poor posture or osteoporosis. The approach to this dysfunction would include prescribed exercises or

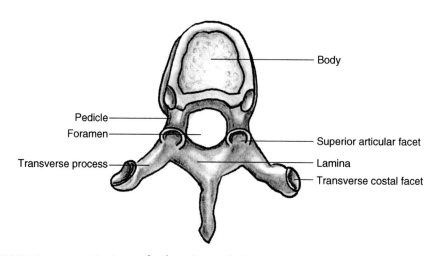

FIGURE 4-19. Anatomy of a thoracic vertebral segment.

physical therapy (PT) to decrease progression of the curve. This may include activity to decrease shoulder protraction such as scapular retractions.

- Flattened thoracic kyphosis generally leads to extension dysfunctions.
- Kyphosis flattens with inhalation and increases with exhalation.
- In general:
  - Flattened kyphosis → inhaled ribs
  - Increased kyphosis → exhaled ribs
- Lateral curves—Group dysfunction—Fryette's Type I—Neutral
  - Fryette's Type I: Sidebent and rotated to opposite sides. Neutral with regard to flexion/extension.
  - A lateral curve is often first detected on a standing structural examination. As the patient bends forward at the waist, a curve may be detected by finding asymmetric **paravertebral humping**. This humping may be because of the rotation of vertebral segments in a group curve. For instance, if one finds paravertebral humping in the right lower thoracic region, this may indicate a group curve, convex right. The vertebral segments are sidebent left and rotated right. The right rotation causes the humping. Alternatively, paravertebral humping may be the result of muscle hypertrophy from a dominant hand and may not be associated with a lateral curve. Motion testing the area would help differentiate these two processes.
  - **Scoliosis**: By definition, a curve is scoliotic if greater than 10°. Measurement of the curve is often done by the Cobb method (See Figure 4-20).
  - Scoliosis is named for the side of the convexity of the curve. In the example above, it would be named right thoracic scoliosis (dextroscoliosis) if it were greater than 10°.
  - Etiology of scoliosis:
    - Idiopathic (majority)
    - Congenital
    - Acquired (short leg and prosthesis)
  - Severity: Surgical intervention is generally indicated in thoracic curves of greater than 50°. Curves greater than this can compromise respiratory and eventually cardiovascular function.
  - Structural versus functional: A functional curve is not yet fixed in place. A heel lift may immediately correct a functional curve, but will not correct a structural curve. As the patient is bent over, humping may

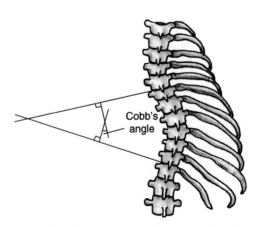

FIGURE 4-20. Cobb method for determining the degree of scoliosis.

decrease in a functional curve as the patient also sidebends. Humping will not decrease in a structural curve with this maneuver.

- Treatment for scoliosis (especially in adults) is generally directed at reducing symptoms created by the curve. Most curves at this age are fixed. The main goal is often to stretch the concave side and to strengthen the convex side to help prevent worsening of the curve. From a segmental standpoint, the apex of the curve and crossover regions can be addressed with segmental techniques such as HVLA, ME, and FPR.
- Segmental dysfunction: Fryette's Type II—Non-neutral
  - Fryette's Type II: One vertebral segment involved, sidebent and rotated to the same side. Non-neutral, meaning there is a component of flexion or extension.
  - Diagnosis of Type II lesions is determined by assessing motion in all three planes (ie, flexion/extension, sidebending, and rotation). A multitude of various approaches to diagnosis exists. Use any that you are comfortable with.

TREATMENT TECHNIQUES

(See Chapter 10.)

- Muscle energy: Thoracic curve, convex left, T3 to T7
- High velocity, low amplitude (Kirksville crunch): T4 extended, rotated left, sidebent left—T4ER$_L$S$_L$
- Counterstrain: Anterior and posterior thoracic tenderpoints

RIBS

RELEVANT ANATOMY

(See Figure 4-21.)

- Head: Articulates with corresponding vertebra and vertebra above it. For example, rib 2 articulates with the superior part of the second vertebral body and the inferior portion of the first vertebral body.
- Neck: Flattened portion between the head and the tuberosity.
- Tubercle: Articulates with transverse process of corresponding vertebra–costotransverse articulation.
- Body or shaft: Portion which extends beyond the tubercle and articulates with the costal cartilage anterior.

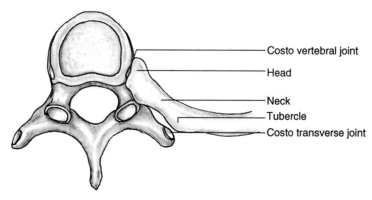

Costo vertebral joint
Head
Neck
Tubercle
Costo transverse joint

FIGURE 4-21. Anatomy of a typical rib.

EXCEPTIONS

- Ribs 1 and 10: Articulate with corresponding vertebra only.
- Ribs 11 and 12: Articulate with corresponding vertebra only. In addition, they have no neck or tubercle and thus no costotransverse articulations.

CLASSIFICATION

- **True ribs** (1-7): Attached to sternum by their costal cartilage
- **False ribs** (8-10): Attached to costal cartilage of ribs above forming anterior costal margin
- **Floating ribs** (11 and 12): No anterior connection, also considered **false ribs** by definition

RIB MOTIONS

Pump Handle Motion

- Predominantly found in upper ribs.
- Anterior aspects of ribs move upward during inspiration.
- Increases anterior-posterior diameter of thorax.

Bucket Handle Motion

- Predominantly found in lower ribs.
- Lateral aspects of the ribs move upward with inspiration.
- Increases transverse diameter of thorax.

Caliper (Pincer Motion)

- Ribs 11 and 12
- External rotation with inspiration

DIAGNOSIS

SD of ribs is typically classified into two groups:

1. Respiratory restrictions
2. Structural dysfunctions

Respiratory Restrictions

- **Inhaled ribs**: Stuck in inhalation, do not move freely into exhalation (Figure 4-22).
- **Exhaled ribs**: Stuck in exhalation, do not move freely into inhalation (Figure 4-23).
- **Key rib**: Often a group of inhaled or exhaled ribs are held restricted by one key rib.

BITE: *Bottom Inhaled, Top Exhaled.*

You can think of the key rib as acting like a dam—it restrains the ribs behind it. So for a group of inhaled ribs, 4 to 6, the bottom rib, sixth, is the key rib. It is stuck in inhalation and doesn't let the ones above it (4 and 5) move into exhalation. Conversely, for a group of exhaled ribs, 7 to 10, the top rib, seventh, is the key rib. It stops the ones below it from going into inhalation. Another way to remember the position of the key rib is the mnemonic **BITE**.

Structural Dysfunctions

- **Anterior ribs**: Prominence and tenderness of rib anteriorly.
- **Posterior ribs**: Prominence of rib angle posteriorly, tenderness and restriction of rib rotation to opposite side.
- **Elevated first rib**: Restriction to inferior motion and when pressing on the posterior aspect of the shaft of the rib. These are commonly very tender.

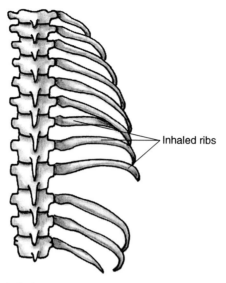

FIGURE 4-22. Inhaled ribs.

TREATMENT TECHNIQUES

Respiratory Restrictions

▪ Muscle energy: Exhaled ribs 1 or 2 on the left

Structural Dysfunctions

▪ Facilitated positional release: Elevated first rib on the left

RESPIRATORY DIAPHRAGM

RELEVANT ANATOMY

(See Figure 4-24.)

ATTACHMENTS

▪ Sternal part: Attached to xyphoid (inner surface)
▪ Costal part: Attached to ribs 7 to 12

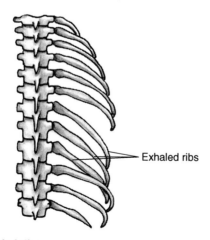

FIGURE 4-23. Exhaled ribs.

Rib angles are often a place where the tenderness and tissue texture change associated with viscerosomatic reflexes are found. To determine if the tissue texture change is caused by a dysfunctional rib or a viscerosomatic response may be difficult. Restriction to motion testing of the rib is evidence for a structural rib dysfunction.

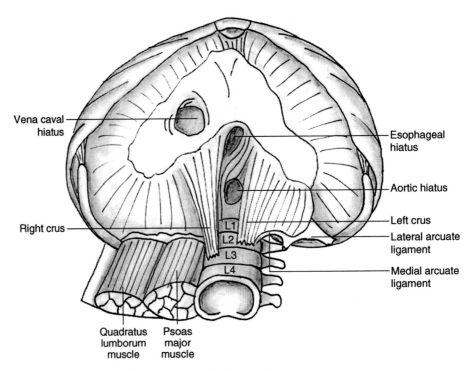

FIGURE 4-24. Anatomy of the respiratory diaphragm.

In addition to its role for lung inflation, the diaphragm also provides a very important pump for venous and lymphatic return. Contraction of the diaphragm during inhalation leads to the descent of the dome. This creates more space in the thoracic region, leading to a negative pressure or vacuum. The contraction also adds pressure to the abdominal cavity. A favorable pressure gradient for fluid return to the thoracic cavity is thus created with each inspiration.

- Lumbar part: Attached to medial and lateral arcuate ligaments (see below)
- Right crus: Attached to bodies of L1 to L3
- Left crus: Attached to bodies of L1 to L2

All of the above insert into the central tendon.

- Medial arcuate ligament: Spans from body of L1 to transverse process of L1
- Lateral arcuate ligament: Spans from transverse process of L1 to rib 12

APERTURES

- T8: Vena caval hiatus in central tendon inferior vena cava (IVC) and right phrenic nerve. Dilates with inspiration allowing venous return
- T10: Esophageal hiatus in muscular part esophagus and vagus nerves. Contracts with inspiration to prevent gastric reflux
- T12: Aortic hiatus between crura aorta, thoracic duct, azygos vein. Not affected by inspiration

DIAGNOSIS

Diagnosis of the diaphragm can be accomplished in many ways. Three common steps are listed:

- Step one: Motion test the diaphragm.
  - Patient seated. Physician behind patient (Figure 4-25).
  - Physician passes his/her arms under patient's arms and around thorax to place fingers under subcostal margin anteriorly.
  - Fingers are slowly advanced up and under ribs as patient leans back into physician and slumps forward.
  - With the patient taking deep breaths, diaphragmatic tension is assessed as the fingers are further advanced up and under the rib cage.

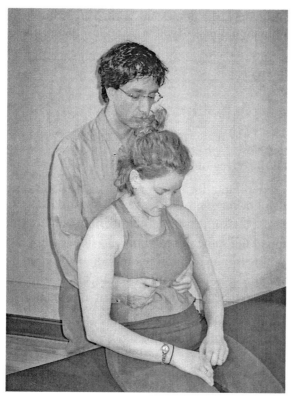

FIGURE 4-25. Diaphragm diagnosis.

- Step two: Check for tight accessory muscles of respiration (scalenes, sternocleidomastoid).
  - Normally these muscles are recruited for breathing with exertion only. Tightness in these muscles may be a result of poor diaphragmatic involvement. Some patients simply do not use their diaphragms well. Often this is secondary to stress.
- Step three: Check for a flattening of the upper lumbar lordosis.
  - Owing to its lumbar attachments, a contracted diaphragm will flatten this curve. This may be assessed visually, by palpation, or by a loss of spring in this region.

TREATMENT TECHNIQUES

- Address a flattened lumbar lordosis if it exists.
- Address myofascial restrictions in chest wall and abdomen.
- Teach the patient abdominal breathing in contrast to accessory muscle use.

(See Chapter 5.)

▶ **REVIEW QUESTIONS: THORACIC/RIBS/DIAPHRAGM DIAGNOSIS**

Questions 1–5

A 43-year-old female comes to your office with a complaint of diffuse back pain which is mostly in the middle of the back. She denies any history of trauma. She denies radicular symptoms. You have seen her several times for urinary tract infections (UTIs), and during this visit, she states that she has again had some pain with urination. She denies any flank pain or history of kidney stones. On physical examination, she is negative for costovertebral angle tenderness.

1. Based on her history, where is the most likely place to find a sympathetic viscerosomatic reflex?
   A. S1 to S2
   B. S2 to S4
   C. C2
   D. T5 to T9
   E. Thoracolumbar region

2. You have found an anterior counterstrain tenderpoint on the left at T10. Which of the following setups is most likely to work?
   A. Extension of the spine, rotation to the right with no sidebending
   B. Extension of the spine, no rotation and sidebending to the right
   C. Flexion of the spine, rotation to the right with no sidebending
   D. Flexion of the spine, sidebending to the left
   E. Spine in neutral, sidebending to the left and rotation to the right

3. You have found a dysfunction in a group of ribs, 7 to 10, on the right. Compared to the left side, these ribs move well with exhalation, but not so well with inhalation. Which of the following best describes this situation?
   A. Inhaled ribs right; seventh rib is the key rib, primarily restricted in bucket handle motion
   B. Exhaled ribs right; seventh rib is the key rib, primarily restricted in bucket handle motion
   C. Exhaled ribs right; tenth rib is the key rib, primarily restricted in pump handle motion
   D. Inhaled ribs right; tenth rib is the key rib, primarily restricted in pump handle motion
   E. Exhaled ribs right; tenth rib is the key rib, primarily restricted in bucket handle motion

4. What additional SD might you expect to find in the region of T7 to T10 for the above patient?
   A. Flattened kyphosis with extended thoracic dysfunctions
   B. Flattened kyphosis with flexed thoracic dysfunctions
   C. Increased kyphosis with extended thoracic dysfunctions
   D. Increased kyphosis with flexed thoracic dysfunctions
   E. Flattened kyphosis with flattened diaphragm

5. You find a dysfunction at the level of T7. The spinous process of T7 can be found at the level of which vertebra?
   A. T5
   B. T6
   C. T7
   D. T8
   E. T9

Questions 6–8

You are performing a standing structural examination on a 24-year-old female who comes to your office with a complaint of back pain and headaches, which she has had intermittently for a number of years. You notice that she has distinct paravertebral humping in the left thoracic region from T3 to T7. Motion testing confirms that a group curve exists, which corresponds to this paravertebral humping.

6. Which of the following best describes the expected findings at T4?
    A. Extended, sidebent right, rotated right
    B. Extended, sidebent left, rotated left
    C. Flexed, sidebent right, rotated right
    D. Flexed, sidebent left, rotated left
    E. Neutral, sidebent right, rotated left

7. The most common measurement or method to determine the degree of curvature on a plain x-ray is by which of the following?
    A. Ferguson angle
    B. Cobb method
    C. Q-angle
    D. Parallax method
    E. Pelvivertebral angle

8. By definition a curve is considered scoliosis if it has a curvature of at least how many degrees?
    A. 5°
    B. 10°
    C. 15°
    D. 20°
    E. 30°

> ANSWERS

Questions 1-5

1, E. 2, D. 3, B. 4, D. 5, D.

Based on her history of UTI, it is reasonable that she has some persistent viscerosomatic reflexes from the bladder. These reflexes may be sympathetic and or parasympathetic. Parasympathetic reflexes for the bladder are found in S2 to S4, but the question asked specifically for sympathetic reflexes. This is the thoracolumbar region for the bladder, answer E. While C2 is a reflex for kidneys and ureters, this again is parasympathetic. Also, her history is more consistent with a UTI than with pyelonephritis or stones; she has no flank pain or costovertebral tenderness and a history of UTIs. For the counterstrain question, you only need to know the general rule that for anterior points it takes flexion and sidebending to the same side (if it is not a midline point), answer D. An exhaled rib is one that goes easily into exhalation. Using the mnemonic BITE, the key rib is the top rib with exhaled ribs, which, in this case, is rib 7. These are lower ribs so they move in a primarily bucket handle motion. In addition, exhaled ribs are often found with an increased kyphosis and flexed thoracic dysfunctions in the area of the exhaled ribs. The spinous process of T7 can be found at the level of T8.

Questions 6–8

6. E, 7. B, 8. B.

T4 is part of the group curve. A group curve follows Freyette's Type I mechanics and so is neutral with respect to flexion and extension. It is also sidebent and rotated to opposite sides. In this case, humping is found on the left, so this is the side of rotation. Only one answer fits this description, answer E. All the other choices follow Type II mechanics. The degree of scoliosis is measured by the Cobb method, answer B. The Ferguson angle is also known as the lumbrosacral angle, answer A. The Q-angle deals with knee mechanics, answer C. The parallax method is used by radiologists to determine the depth of objects on films, answer D. The pelvivertebral angle measures the tilt of the pelvis with respect to the spinal column, answer E. And finally, scoliosis is defined by a curve of at least 10°, answer B.

Relevant Anatomy

BONY

(See Figure 4-26.)

- Five lumbar vertebrae.
- Facets angled toward the sagittal plane; allows for maximum flexion and extension.
- Normal lumbar curve is lordotic.
- Large vertebral bodies. Long, slender transverse processes point laterally. Round, blunted, spinous processes point posteriorly.

MUSCULAR

ERECTOR SPINAE

Superficial Back Muscles

- Iliocostalis, Longissimus, and Spinalis (I Like Spaghetti)
- Primarily extend spine
- Also sidebend and rotate to ipsilateral side

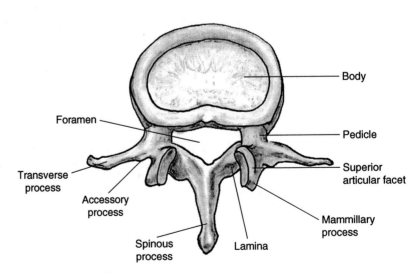

FIGURE 4-26. Lumbar vertebrae.

MULTIFIDUS

Deep Back Muscles

- Predominant in the lumbar region
- Extend and sidebend to the ipsilateral side
- Rotate to the opposite side

PSOAS

- Originates on the anterior aspect of vertebrae T12 to L5
- Combines with the iliacus (to form the iliopsoas complex)
- Inserts on lesser trochanter of the femur
- Flexes hip. If feet are fixed, flexes trunk. Also laterally flexes vertebral column to the ipsilateral side
- Major pelvic stabilizer, tonically contracted while standing
- Extremely common source of low back pain

QUADRATES LUMBORUM

- Originates on the iliac crest and iliolumbar ligament
- Inserts on inferior aspect of the twelfth rib, as well as transverse processes of vertebrae 1 to 4
- Extends the vertebral column with bilateral extension and fixes the twelfth rib during inspiration
- Major stabilizer of the pelvic girdle

RESPIRATORY DIAPHRAGM

(See Diagnosis for Thoracic Spine.)

LIGAMENTOUS

- The iliolumbar ligament originates on the iliac crest and inserts on the transverse processes of L4 to L5.
- Results in decreased mobility of L4 and L5 compared to the upper three lumbar vertebrae.
- Dysfunction of the iliolumbar ligament can produce a wide array of referred pain patterns.

NERVOUS

- Spinal cord typically ends near the L2 level (and continues as the cauda equina).
- Preganglionic sympathetic cell bodies are found in upper lumbar segments of the spinal cord (L1-L2).
- Afferent pain stimulus travels along sympathetic fibers to spinal cord via white rami communicantes. White rami communicantes are found in the upper thoracic levels and terminate at the upper lumbar levels.
- Several nerves of the lumbar plexus pass in close proximity to the iliopsoas complex.
- The genitofemoral nerve passes directly through psoas major muscle; therefore, psoas tension can cause anterior thigh or groin symptoms.

Diagnosis

Many disease processes can cause low back pain. The history and physical examination help identify the pain as neurological, musculoskeletal, arthritic, inflammatory, and so on.

The deep back muscles contain more muscle spindles (which sense stretch) and sensory innervation than the larger, superficial back muscles. In addition, they are more likely to become strained. With this combination they are likely a significant cause of musculoskeletal back pain.

Remember that a hypertonic psoas muscle is associated with "flexed" lumbar dysfunction. Lumbar segments are sidebent to the side of the hypertonic psoas and rotated away from the side of the hypertonic psoas.

Diagnosis of the lumbar spine for SD involves active and passive range of motion and a standing structural examination (ie, screening for group curves, single segment motion, psoas evaluation, seated flexion test, and standing flexion test). If sacroiliac (SI) dysfunction is present, chances are lumbar SD is present as well.

(See section on sacrum and pelvis diagnosis for more on lumbosacral junction.)

The lumbar spine may exhibit either Type I or II mechanics.

TYPE I MECHANICS

- Often because of a short leg, scoliosis, or a unilaterally tight psoas.

(See Thoracic Diagnosis for more on scoliosis.)

SHORT LEG MECHANICS

- Two types: Functional and anatomical.
- A functional short leg commonly results from discord between myofascial forces. A functional short leg is identical in length to its counterpart, but "functions" as a shorter extremity as a result of altered muscle tone, fascial restriction, or postural imbalance.
- Anatomical short leg is typically congenital (usually a bony problem) or a result of surgical intervention.
- An anatomical short leg is physically shorter than its counterpart secondary to fracture, deformity, or altered growth.

FUNCTIONAL SHORT LEG

(See Figure 4-27.)

- Length discrepancy causes sacral base unleveling and pelvic sideshift to the long leg side, allowing the long leg to burden the added weight of the trunk.
- A lumbar group curve develops convex to the short leg side.
- The sacrum sidebends **toward** the short leg side and rotates **away**. The sacrum rotates and sidebends in opposite directions as it does in a forward torsion. The sacrum leaves a deep sulcus on the short leg side.
- The seated flexion test will be positive on the short leg side.

(See Table 4-2 for further anatomic findings related to a short leg.)

ANATOMICAL SHORT LEG

- Anatomical short legs cause patterns similar to those found with functional short legs. However, the patterns result from bones that are physically shorter than one another. Anatomical short legs, if diagnosed early in life or immediately after surgery, can be treated effectively with a heel lift. Anatomical short legs, if left untreated for a long period of time, can develop SD that is very difficult to treat.

TYPE II MECHANICS

- Related to single segment dysfunction.
- Flexed, sidebent, and rotated to the same side. Often found with a decreased lordosis of the lumbar spine.

Anterior innominate rotation will functionally lengthen the leg on the side of rotation. Conversely, a posterior innominate rotation functionally shortens the same leg.

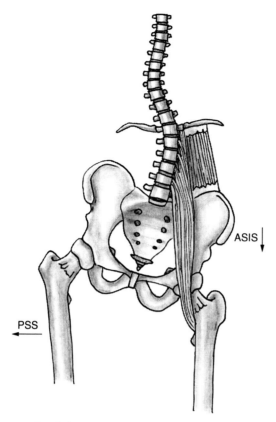

FIGURE 4-27. Functional short leg.

TABLE 4-2. Manifestations of a Short Leg

STRUCTURE	MANIFESTATION
Lumbar spine	Convex on short leg side
Sacral sulcus	Deep on short leg side
Sacral ILA	Posterior on long leg side
Innominate	Anterior on short leg side
Psoas	Hypertonic on short leg side
Quadratus	Hypertonic on short leg side
Piriformis	Hypertonic on long leg side
Gluteus medius	Hypertonic on short leg side

ILA, inferior lateral angle.

- Flexed upper lumbar dysfunctions are associated with a hypertonic psoas. You may find a flexed lumbar segment rotated and sidebent to side of the hypertonic psoas.
- Extended, sidebent, and rotated to the same side. Common with an increased lumbar lordosis.

In addition to SD, there are several anatomic variations that, when present, can produce low back pain.

SACRALIZATION OF L5

- L5 fuses either partially or completely with the sacrum. This causes limited motion at the lumbosacral junction.

LUMBARIZATION OF S1

- S1 fails to fuse with the remainder of the sacrum. This results in greater mobility at the lumbosacral junction, which may lead to instability in this region.

BAT WING DEFORMITY

- Results from enlargement of the transverse processes of L5. This may lead to limited motion at the lumbosacral junction.

SPONDYLOLYSIS

On x-ray, spondylolysis appears as a "collar" on a "Scottie dog."

- Fracture of the pars interarticularis. May happen unilaterally or bilaterally. If bilateral, results in forward slippage of the anterior aspect of the vertebrae (Figure 4-28).

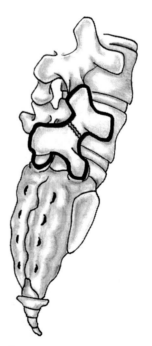

FIGURE 4-28. The Scottie dog.

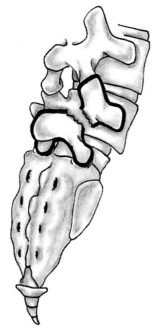

FIGURE 4-29. Spondylolisthesis.

SPONDYLOLISTHESIS

- Anterior slippage of one vertebra in relation to the vertebrae below (often occurs at L5 on S1). Graded according to the percentage of slippage (Figure 4-29)
- Grade 1: 1% to 25%
- Grade 2: 26% to 50%
- Grade 3: 51% to 75%
- Grade 4: 76% to 100%

SPINAL STENOSIS

- Narrowing of the intervertebral foramina causes nerve root irritation and radicular symptoms.

HERNIATED DISC

- Caused by a tear in the annulus fibrosis. Irritation to the nerve root exiting below the disc is caused by mechanical compression or chemical irritation from the nucleus pulposus. Example: An L4 nerve root is irritated by the L3 disc.

Treatment Techniques

(See Chapter 10.)

- High velocity, low amplitude: Lateral recumbent for Type II dysfunction, T10 to L5
- Counterstrain: Anterior L1 to L5 (AL1-AL5)
- Counterstrain: Posterior L1 to L5 (PL1-PL5)

- Facilitated positional release: Flexed SD
- Facilitated positional release: Extended SD
- High velocity, low amplitude: Leg pull dysfunction: Short leg
- Muscle energy: Psoas muscle spasm

Questions 1–5

A 34-year-old male presents to the clinic with a 2-day history of low back pain after traveling 8 hours in the car recently. The pain is focal, bilateral, dull, and constant. After a negative workup, you decide to treat this patient using OMT.

1. On examination, you notice the seated flexion test is positive on the right, pelvic sideshift is positive left, and the lumbar spine has a decreased lordosis. The sacrum is rotated to the left on a left oblique axis. What muscle do you suspect is contributing to these findings?
   A. Hypertonic psoas on the right
   B. Hypertonic psoas on the left
   C. Hypertonic iliocostalis on the right
   D. Hypertonic iliocostalis on the left
   E. Hypertonic multifidus on the left

2. What other SD might you expect to find in the upper lumbar segments?
   A. Extended, rotated right, sidebent right
   B. Extended, rotated left, sidebent left
   C. Flexed, rotated right, sidebent right
   D. Flexed, rotated left, sidebent left
   E. Flexed, rotated left, sidebent right

3. You note the patient has an anterior counterstrain tenderpoint at the area corresponding to L1. Where would you monitor this point when treating with counterstrain?
   A. Over the anterior superior iliac spine (ASIS)
   B. Over the medial aspect of the anterior inferior iliac spine (AIIS)
   C. Over the lateral aspect of the AIIS
   D. Over the umbilicus
   E. Over the pubic tubercle

4. To treat the above point using counterstrain, how is the patient positioned?
   A. Prone
   B. Supine
   C. On the left side
   D. On the right side
   E. Seated

5. The patient also complains of anterior thigh and groin pain. What nerve would you suspect is irritated?
   A. Iliohypogastric
   B. Ilioinguinal
   C. Subcostal
   D. Genitofemoral
   E. Obturator

A 25-year-old female patient presents to you with back pain after a motor vehicle accident (MVA) that she was involved in 4 months ago. The pain is focal, dull, greater on the right than the left, and worse with physical activity. Previously, she has never complained of any such pain, nor has she worn any type of orthotic or heel lift. After a negative workup, you decide to treat her using OMT. Answer the following questions in order.

6. On examination, you notice that the seated flexion test is positive on the left, pelvic side shift is positive on the right, and the lumbar spine has a group curve that is convex to the left. What is your initial impression?
   A. Gluteus medius hypertonicity on the right
   B. Psoas hypertonicity on the right
   C. Piriformis hypertonicity on the left
   D. Posterior innominate on the right
   E. Short leg on the left

7. After you have completed your full osteopathic examination, you conclude that she has a short leg. Given the patient's history and physical findings, do you suspect this to be a(n)
   A. Anatomical short leg on the left
   B. Anatomical short leg on the right
   C. Functional short leg on the left
   D. Functional short leg on the right
   E. Both functional and anatomical short leg on the left

8. Which way would sacral sidebending and rotation occur in this patient?
   A. Sidebent to the left, rotated to the right
   B. Sidebent to the right, rotated to the left
   C. Sidebent to the right, rotated to the right
   D. Sidebent to the left, no rotation of the sacrum
   E. Sidebent to the right, no rotation of the sacrum

9. After further evaluation, you also notice that her left ASIS is superior in relation to her right ASIS. What would you also then include in the objective portion of your subjective, objective, assessment, plan (SOAP) note? That the patient has a(n)
   A. Posterior innominate on the right
   B. Anterior innominate on the right
   C. Anterior innominate on the left
   D. Posterior innominate on the left
   E. None of the above

10. You decide to treat this patient's posterior innominate on the left with ME. Which of the following best describes the key forces involved in this treatment technique?
    A. You exert a force to extend the patient's hip (into the barrier) while they exert a counterforce against you to flex their hip (away from the barrier).
    B. You exert a force to flex the patient's hip (away from the barrier) while they exert a counterforce against you to extend their hip (into the barrier).
    C. You exert a force to extend the patient's hip (into the barrier) while they exert an additional force with you to extend their hip further (into the barrier).

D. You exert a force to flex the patient's hip (away from the barrier) while they exert an additional force with you to flex their hip (into the barrier).
E. A posterior innominate cannot be treated with ME.
F. Muscle energy techniques are contraindicated in this patient.

▶ ANSWERS

1. A

Given the sideshift, sacral motion, and decreased lordosis, you should suspect a psoas issue on the right side as a contributing factor. Remember, a tight psoas compresses the SI joint and lumbar spine on that side. Therefore, you may get a lumbar convexity on that side. If the convexity is on the right, the sacrum will sidebend to the right to accommodate the curve. The sacrum rotates and sidebends to opposite sides; therefore, it will rotate to the left on a left oblique axis. Regardless, neither a tight iliocostalis nor multifidus should produce this constellation of findings.

2. C

A tight psoas may result in a flexed upper lumbar Type II lesion. Typically, you will find a flexed segment rotated and sidebent to the side of the tight psoas.

3. A

According to *Foundations of Osteopathic Medicine*, the anterior lumbar tenderpoints are located as follows: **AL1**: medial side of ASIS, press laterally; **AL2**: medial side of AIIS, press laterally; **AL3**: lateral side of AIIS, press medially; **AL4**: inferior side of AIIS, press cephalad; **AL5**: anterior surface of pubic rami approximately 1 cm lateral to pubic symphysis and inferior to tubercle, press posteriorly.

4. B

Treatment of anterior lumbar tenderpoints occurs with the patient supine.

5. D

While several nerves from the lumbar plexus pass in close proximity to the psoas muscle, the genitofemoral nerve actually passes through the belly of the muscle itself. Therefore, of the above nerves, the genitofemoral nerve is the most likely to cause this patient's symptoms.

6. E

Given the sideshift, seated flexion test, and lumbar group curve, you should suspect a short leg on the left. Choices A through C are all manifestations of a short leg, but not on the left. They refer to manifestations of a short leg on the right. A posterior innominate on the right would cause a short leg on the right, not the left. Go back and review Table 4-2.

7. C

As stated above for question number 6, you should already know that she has a short leg on the left. To clue you in that it is a functional short leg, there is one important clue you can take a look at. She is 25 years old, and has just started complaining of back pain after an MVA. She did not have any previous back pain before the accident; it was only after the trauma occurred that the pain presented. Furthermore, she has never worn any heel lift which would correct a leg length inequality. Heel lifts are usually prescribed for anatomical short legs, whereas treating the cause of the short leg is the prescription for functional short legs.

8. A

The sacrum would be sidebent to the left and rotated to the right. For both anatomical and functional short legs, the sacrum always sidebends to the short leg side. Since the sacrum rotates and sidebends in opposite directions, the sacrum will rotate away from the short leg (to the right) leaving a deep sulcus on the short leg side (on the left).

9. D

Innominate rotation can also vary leg length. An anterior innominate lengthens the leg, while a posterior innominate shortens the leg. To determine whether it is an anterior innominate on the right versus a posterior innominate on the left, use the side of the seated flexion test. Since the seated flexion test was on the left (will always be positive on the side of the short leg), then the innominate diagnosis is a posterior innominate on the left.

10. A

If you would like to treat the patient with ME, you need to introduce a counterforce against the patient into the barrier. Conversely, the patient will exert a force away from the barrier. This general concept holds true for all ME techniques. Since the innominate is rotated posteriorly, you will bring it into an anterior position. Extending the patient's hip results in bringing the patient's innominate into this anterior position.

► SACRUM AND PELVIS DIAGNOSIS

Sacrum

RELEVANT ANATOMY

- Formed from five fused vertebrae (Figure 4-30).
- The sacrum has two L-shaped articulations it shares with the ilium (Figure 4-31).
- The sacrum glides along this L-shaped articulation.

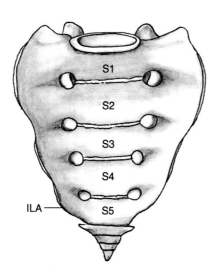

FIGURE 4-30. Sacrum—anterior view.

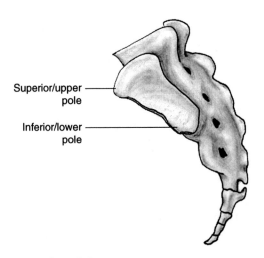

Superior/upper
pole

Inferior/lower
pole

FIGURE 4-31. Sacrum—lateral view.

REGIONAL AND SYSTEMS-
BASED ASSESSMENT

REGIONAL DIAGNOSIS

*CRAIN—from superior to
inferior—Cranial/Respiratory
Anatomical Innominate.*

UNIQUE TERMINOLOGY

- **Nutation**: The sacral base moves anteriorly and inferiorly while the sacral apex moves posteriorly and superiorly.
- **Counternutation**: The sacral base moves posteriorly and superiorly while the sacral apex moves anteriorly and inferiorly.

SACRAL MOTION

- The sacrum moves about three transverse axes: superior, middle, and inferior (Figure 4-32).
- **Superior transverse axis**: Site of respiratory or craniosacral flexion and or extension of the sacrum.
- **Middle transverse axis**: Site of anatomical sacral flexion and extension.
- **Inferior transverse axis**: Site of innominate motion on the sacrum.
- **Oblique Axes**: Physiological axes created as a result of changes in weight bearing. These axes run from the superior pole/articular surface

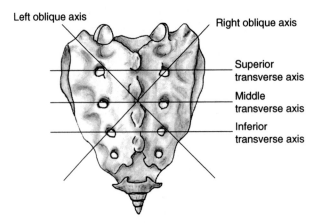

Left oblique axis

Right oblique axis

Superior
transverse axis

Middle
transverse axis

Inferior
transverse axis

FIGURE 4-32. Sacrum—posterior view with axes.

74

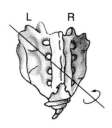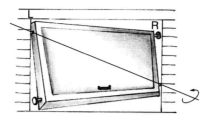

FIGURE 4-33. Sacral motion about a left oblique axis.

on one side of the sacrum to the inferior pole/articular surface on the opposite side of the sacrum. There are two oblique axes: right and left. The oblique axis is named for the superior aspect of the sacrum of which the axis travels.

- To get a better handle on sacral rotation about the oblique axes, think of the sacrum like a garage door. The two superior corners of the garage door are the sacral sulci, while the two inferior corners of the garage door are the inferior lateral angle (ILA) of the sacrum (Figure 4-33).
- The garage door glides in two L-shaped tracks on either side, just like the sacrum glides in two L-shaped articulations.
- Now, think of a garage door that gets jammed such that the superior left and the inferior right corner of the garage door get stuck. Meanwhile, the superior right corner and inferior left corner come off the tracks.
- Since the superior left and inferior right corners cannot move, if the door starts to fall forward at the top, the superior right corner falls forward, while the inferior left corner moves toward you. The "jammed" aspects of the garage door are equivalent to the "engaged" axis of the sacrum and the left oblique axis is engaged.
- Now replace the garage door with a sacrum. The right sulcus is deep or anterior (away from you), while the left ILA is posterior (toward you). The sacrum is named for the anterior superior aspect of the bone (as is any vertebrae); therefore, the sacrum is rotated to the left.

Remember, the oblique axis is named for the superior aspect of the sacrum through which it travels.

DIAGNOSIS

Diagnosis and treatment of the sacrum is a favorite topic on boards. One difficulty with this area is the different terminologies used to describe sacral dysfunction at different osteopathic medical schools. Two main types of frameworks exist to describe sacral mechanics: sacral torsions and the anterior/posterior sacrum model. The majority of osteopathic schools teach the torsion model. However, the anterior/posterior sacral model is the primary model for a minority of osteopathic schools; therefore it is included here. The main point to keep in mind is not to confuse the two models. They are separate because the reference point is different for each of them.

One way questions on boards avoid this issue is by focusing on sacral motion about the oblique axes, which is common to both frameworks. Therefore, the goal with any sacral question should be to establish which direction the sacrum is moving about which oblique axis; for example, rotated right about a right oblique axis. From there, any further information needed to answer a sacrum board question can usually be obtained easily.

Once the direction of sacral rotation and the axis are determined, you should be able to answer almost any sacrum question regardless of which model you learned.

SACRAL TORSION MODEL

- The most common model used to describe sacral mechanics.
- The point of reference for this model is the sacrum in relation to L5. Therefore, all sacral diagnoses are named in reference to L5.
- Torsion means twisting. In a sacral torsion, the sacrum is *always* rotated in the opposite direction of L5 (Figure 4-34).
- It is helpful to think about diagnosis of the sacrum in this model following a specific set of steps. The typical test question will provide information about some of these steps, then require you fill in the remaining blanks in order to answer the question.
- **Step one: Diagnose L5.**
  - This is a crucial step for diagnosing sacral torsions. The diagnosis of L5 will determine whether you have a forward or backward torsion.
  - If L5 is in neutral mechanics, you will have a forward torsion.
  - If L5 is in non-neutral mechanics, you will have a backward torsion.
  - The side to which L5 is sidebent determines the axis about which the sacrum rotates. For example, if L5 is sidebent left, the left oblique axis is engaged (the garage door is jammed on the superior left side) (Figures 4-33 and 4-35).
- **Step two: Seated flexion test.**
  - The seated flexion test indicates there is SI dysfunction on the side of a positive test.
  - A negative test indicates two things: (1) There is no SI dysfunction. (2) The test is actually falsely negative, meaning the SI joints are restricted bilaterally. This happens with bilateral sacral flexions and extensions.
  - With torsion, the seated flexion test will be positive on the side *opposite* the engaged oblique axis. For example, in a forward torsion rotated right on a right oblique axis, the seated flexion test will be positive on the left.
- **Step three: Check sulcus depth.**
  - Determine which sulcus is deeper. Remember, forward torsions result in a deep sulcus on the opposite side of the engaged axis. Backward torsions result in a shallow sulcus on the opposite side of the engaged axis.

The point of reference for the torsion model is the sacrum in relation to L5.

Remember Fryette's principles: **Type I mechanics** *= the spine is in neutral; rotation and sidebending occur to opposite sides.* **Type II mechanics** *= the spine is in non-neutral (flexion or extension); rotation and sidebending occur to the same side.*

*One **N** Forward, Two **N**s Back Neutral = forward torsion Non-neutral backward torsion.*

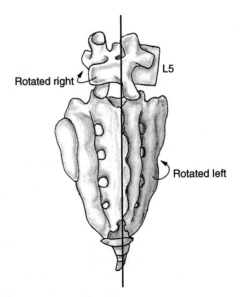

Rotated right

L5

Rotated left

FIGURE 4-34. Rotation component of sacral torsion.

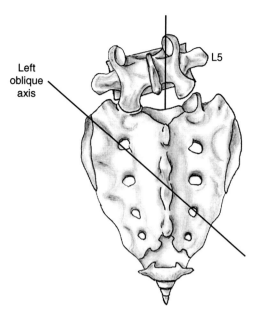

Left
oblique
axis

L5

FIGURE 4-35. **Sidebending component of sacral torsion.**

Sulcus asymmetry rules out a bilateral sacral flexion or extension. In addition, forward torsions are typically symptomatic (increased tissue texture change and tenderness) over the deep sulcus, while backward torsions are typically symptomatic over the shallow sulcus.

- **Step four: Check for posterior ILA.**
  - This step rules in or out the less common sacral dysfunctions, like sacral flexions and extensions. For example, if the posterior ILA is on the *same* side as a deep sulcus, you have a unilateral sacral dysfunction. If the posterior ILA is on the *opposite* side of the deep sulcus, you know you will have a forward or backward torsion. See below for more on other sacral diagnoses.
- **Step five: Determine type of sacral rotation and oblique axis.**
  - This should be the goal of each sacral board question. Using the above first four steps, you should be able to come up with a diagnosis. However, it is critical to think about the diagnosis in terms of rotation about an oblique axis in this model, as this is what board questions commonly ask.
  - Remember, the *sidebending* of L5 determines the *axis* that is engaged (same side).
  - The *rotation* of L5 determines the *rotation* of the sacrum (opposite direction).
  - The *seated flexion test* will be positive on the side opposite the engaged oblique axis.
  - Knowing if you have a forward or backward torsion helps determine the type of rotation and axis.
  - Forward torsions are *always* rotated right about a right axis or rotated left about a left axis (rotated *forward* on the axis).
  - Backward torsions are *always* rotated right about a left axis or rotated left about a right axis (rotated *backward* on the axis).

Two additional tests you may see on boards are the lumbosacral spring test and the backward bending (or sphinx) test.

The sidebending of L5 determines which oblique axis is engaged.

WARNING: Some test questions will not describe a shallow sulcus. Instead, they will describe the sulcus opposite a shallow sulcus as being "deep." For example, a shallow sulcus on the right will be described as a deep sulcus on the left. The left sulcus is not necessarily deep; it is just deep relative to the right sulcus.

If L5 is sidebent left and rotated right, you suspect you have a forward torsion (neutral mechanics). The left oblique axis is engaged (sidebent left) and the sacrum is rotated to the left (L5 is rotated right); therefore, the sacrum is rotated left on a left oblique axis.

*Remember the steps involved
with diagnosing torsions:
Diagnosing Sacral Torsions
Sucks Immensely. Diagnose
L5, Seated flexion Test, Sulcus
depth, ILA.*

*Lumbosacral Spring Test Hint:
Negative = normal (normal
lordotic curve) Positive =
pathology (reversed lordotic
curve).*

*Backward Bending/Sphinx
Test Hint: Forward torsion–
sulcus asymmetry improves
backward torsion––sulcus
asymmetry worsens*

LUMBOSACRAL SPRING TEST

▪ This information helps confirm whether you are dealing with a forward or backward torsion. In the absence of information regarding L5, this can be the only information you receive about the lumbar spine. If you are given information about L5 and the lumbosacral spring test, you should already suspect you are dealing with a forward or backward torsion.

▪ This test is performed by pressing anteriorly on the lumbosacral junction with the patient in the prone position.

▪ A *positive* test indicates *no* spring at the lumbosacral junction. This means the sacrum is in relative extension while L5 is in relative flexion. This is suggestive of a backward torsion, unilateral sacral extension, or bilateral sacral extension.

▪ A *negative* test indicates there is spring at the lumbosacral junction. Therefore, the sacrum is in relative flexion, while L5 is in relative extension. This is a normal finding but may also be suggestive of a forward torsion, unilateral sacral flexion, or bilateral sacral flexion.

▪ A *positive* lumbosacral spring test is abnormal. Normally, the lumbar spine is lordotic, and pressing on the lumbosacral junction should provide some "give." If the sacrum is extended (counternutation) and L5 is flexed, this lordotic curve is reversed. Therefore, pressing on the lumbosacral junction provides no "give" (Figure 4-36).

BACKWARD BENDING/SPHINX TEST

▪ A patient lying prone is asked to extend their back and rest on their elbows (see Figure 4-37). In a *forward* torsion, the sulcus *asymmetry improves* (more symmetrical). In a *backward* torsion, the sulcus *asymmetry worsens* (less symmetrical).

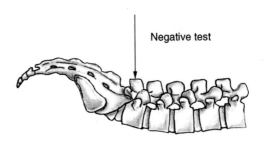

Negative test

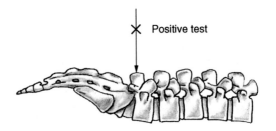

Positive test

FIGURE 4-36. Lumbosacral spring test.

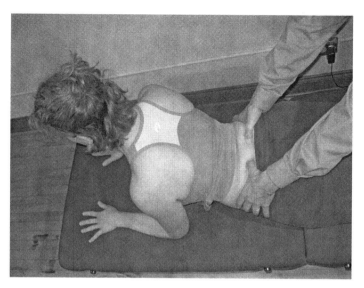

FIGURE 4-37. Backward bending/sphinx test.

EXAMPLE 1

- **Step one:** L5 is in neutral mechanics, sidebent right, and rotated left. This gives you a lot of information. You suspect a forward torsion. The right oblique axis should be engaged (because L5 is sidebent right), and the sacrum should be rotated to the right (because L5 is rotated left and the sacrum rotates opposite L5 in the sacral torsion model).
- **Step two:** Seated flexion test is positive on the left. This goes along with an engaged right oblique axis. A positive test also rules out a bilateral sacral dysfunction.
- **Step three:** There is a deep sulcus on the left. This helps confirm the sacrum is rotated to the right, although there could still be a unilateral sacral dysfunction. The sulcus asymmetry also rules out a bilateral sacral dysfunction.
- **Step four:** The right ILA is posterior. This rules out a unilateral sacral dysfunction.
- **Step five:** The posterior right ILA confirms the sacrum is rotated to the right on a right oblique axis. The diagnosis is a right on right forward torsion (Figure 4-38).

EXAMPLE 2

- **Step one:** L5 is flexed, rotated right, and sidebent right. This tells us we most likely have a backward torsion. The right oblique axis should be engaged (because L5 is sidebent right), and the sacrum should be rotated to the left (because L5 is rotated to the right and the sacrum rotates opposite L5 in the sacral torsion model).
- **Step two:** Seated flexion test is positive on the left. This fits with an engaged right oblique axis.
- **Step three:** The right sulcus is deep. Keep in mind, all this means is the right sulcus is deeper than the left. Therefore, we could interpret this to mean the left sulcus is shallow. This fits with our presumptive diagnosis of a backward torsion, rotated to the left on a right oblique axis. Additionally, the sulcus asymmetry rules out a bilateral sacral dysfunction.
- **Step four:** The left ILA is posterior. This rules out a unilateral sacral dysfunction, as the deeper sulcus and posterior ILA are on opposite sides.
- **Step five:** As we suspected, we have a backward torsion, rotated to the left on a right oblique axis (Figure 4-39).

Hint: You will also have a positive lumbosacral spring test in a backward torsion. The positive lumbosacral spring test helps to rule out a unilateral/bilateral sacral flexion.

79

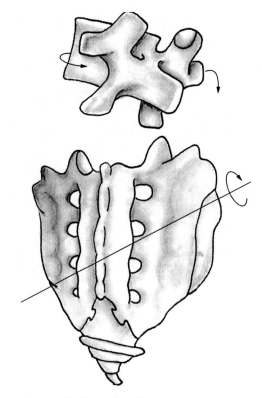

FIGURE 4-38.   Right on right forward torsion.

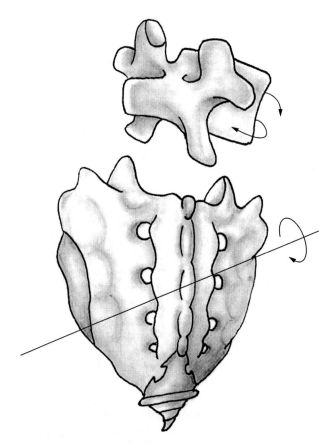

FIGURE 4-39.   Left on right backward torsion.

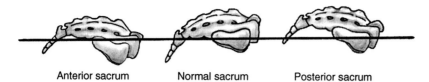

Anterior sacrum   Normal sacrum   Posterior sacrum

FIGURE 4-40. Anterior, normal, and posterior sacrum.

ANTERIOR/POSTERIOR SACRUM MODEL

- The point of reference for this model is the sacrum in relation to the *innominate*. Therefore, all sacral diagnoses are named in reference to the innominate. An anterior sacrum is *anterior* to the innominate. A posterior sacrum is *posterior* to the innominate (Figure 4-40).
- As with the torsion model, diagnosis of the sacrum in this model follows a specific set of steps. Some of this information will be given in the questions. You must then determine the diagnosis and motion about the oblique axis.
- **Step one: Seated flexion test.**
  - This test is the *first* step to diagnose the sacrum in this model. This tells you which side of the sacrum the dysfunction is on. Period. It tells you *nothing* about the type of dysfunction.
- **Step two: Check sulcus depth.**
  - Determine which sulcus is deeper. Sulcus asymmetry also rules out bilateral sacral flexions and extensions.
- **Step three: Check for posterior ILA.**
  - This step rules in or out unilateral sacral flexions and extensions. For example, if the posterior ILA is on the *same* side as a deep sulcus, you have a unilateral dysfunction. If the ILA is on the *opposite* side of the deep sulcus, you know you have an anterior or posterior sacrum.
- **Step four: Determine area of greatest tissue texture change.**
  - If the greatest area of tissue texture change is over the deep sulcus, you have an anterior sacrum on that side. If there is tissue texture change over the posterior ILA, you have a posterior sacrum on that side.
  - "What if the seated flexion test is positive right, there is a deep sulcus on the right, but the area of tissue texture change is over the posterior ILA on the left?" This could happen clinically, but is avoided on boards, as it would confuse everyone.
  - In bilateral sacral flexions and extension, there will be tissue texture changes bilaterally.
- **Step five: Determine type of sacral rotation and oblique axis.**
  - Again, using the above four steps, you should be able to come up with a diagnosis. However, it is critical to think about the diagnosis in terms of rotation about an oblique axis, as this is what board questions commonly ask.
  - In the anterior/posterior sacrum model, this step is actually quite easy (See examples below). Since backward rotation about an oblique axis (ie, backward torsions) are not described in this model, there is *never* right rotation about a left oblique axis or left rotation about a right oblique axis.

EXAMPLE 1

- **Step one:** Seated flexion test is positive on the *right*. This tells you the problem is on the right, nothing else. It could be an anterior sacrum on the right, a posterior sacrum on the right, or a unilateral dysfunction on the right.

Hint: The point of reference for the anterior/posterior sacrum model is the sacrum in relation to the innominates.

One difference between this model and the torsion model is once you know the rotation and axis of the sacrum there are two possible diagnoses. For example, if the sacrum is rotated right on a right oblique axis, you either have an anterior left or posterior right dysfunction. Use the seated flexion test to determine which one is present.

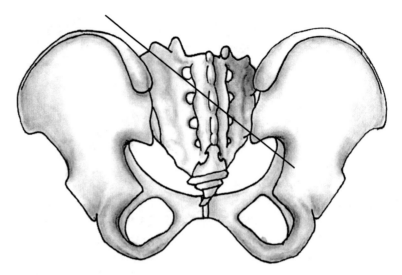

FIGURE 4-41. Right anterior sacrum.

*Remember the steps involved with diagnosing an anterior or posterior sacrum. Using the mnemonic **SSIT**. You **SSIT** on your sacrum. **S**eated flexion test, **S**ulcus depth, **I**LA, **T**issue texture change.*

The main component that differentiates the two models is information about L5. If diagnostic information about L5 is given in the question stem, it will usually be a question pertaining to torsions. Confused? Use the questions at the end of the chapter to help clarify these concepts.

- **Step two:** The right sulcus is deeper. This tells you that you either have an anterior sacrum on the right or a unilateral dysfunction on the right. The sulcus asymmetry rules out a bilateral sacral dysfunction.
- **Step three:** The left ILA is posterior. This rules out a unilateral dysfunction.
- **Step four:** There is increased tissue texture change over the deep sulcus on the right. This determines our diagnosis—anterior sacrum on the right.
- **Step five:** Finally, if we have an anterior sacrum on the right, we know the sacrum is rotated to the left about a left oblique axis (Figure 4-41).

EXAMPLE 2

- **Step one:** Seated flexion test is positive on the *right*. Again, this tells you the problem is on the right, nothing else. It could be an anterior sacrum on the right, a posterior sacrum on the right, or a unilateral dysfunction on the right.
- **Step two:** The left sulcus is deeper. This rules out an anterior sacrum on the right. This tells you there is either a posterior sacrum on the right or a unilateral dysfunction on the right. The sulcus asymmetry rules out a bilateral sacral dysfunction.
- **Step three:** The right ILA is posterior. This rules out a unilateral dysfunction.
- **Step four:** There is tissue texture change over the right ILA. This determines our diagnosis—posterior sacrum on the right.
- **Step five:** Finally, if we have a posterior sacrum on the right, we know the sacrum is rotated right on a right oblique axis (Figure 4-42).

OTHER SACRAL DIAGNOSES: SACRAL FLEXIONS AND EXTENSIONS

- Four types: Unilateral sacral flexion, bilateral sacral flexion, unilateral sacral extension, bilateral sacral extension.
- Not as commonly emphasized on boards.
- Occur when either one or both sides of the sacrum anatomically flex or extend along the L-shaped articulation about the superior (unilateral) or middle (bilateral) transverse axes and get stuck that way. Therefore, no oblique axes are engaged in these dysfunctions.

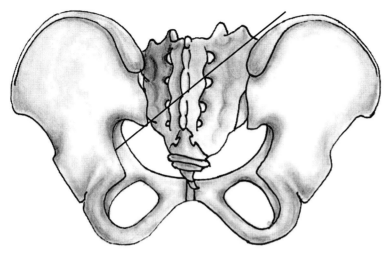

FIGURE 4-42. Right posterior sacrum.

- Findings:
  - Unilateral/bilateral sacral flexion = negative spring test (good spring).
  - Unilateral/bilateral sacral extension = positive spring test (no spring).
  - Unilateral sacral flexion/extension = seated flexion test is positive on side of dysfunction.
  - Unilateral sacral flexion/extension = tissue texture changes on side of dysfunction.
  - Diagnosis of unilateral dysfunctions is made when the posterior ILA is on the *same* side as the deep sulcus.
  - Bilateral sacral flexion/extension = seated flexion test is falsely negative (actually positive bilaterally, so both posterior superior iliac spines [PSIS] rise symmetrically).
  - Bilateral sacral flexion/extension = tissue texture changes bilaterally.
  - Bilateral sacral flexion = ILAs will be posterior bilaterally.
  - Bilateral sacral extension = ILAs will be anterior bilaterally.
- If no information about the lumbosacral spring test is given, differentiation between bilateral sacral flexion and extension is made by motion testing the sacrum in flexion and extension. Bilateral sacral flexion will resist extension of the sacrum, while bilateral sacral extension will resist sacral flexion. Either the lumbosacral spring test or sacral motion testing must be given in a question in order to differentiate between these two types of dysfunctions. Remember, in a bilateral sacral dysfunction, the seated flexion test will be equal bilaterally, sulcus depth will be equal bilaterally, ILA position will be equal bilaterally, and tissue texture change will be equal bilaterally.

*Remember: A seated flexion test can be **falsely negative** indicating **bilateral** sacral dysfunction.*

The posterior ILA is on the same side of the deep sulcus in a unilateral sacral dysfunction.

TREATMENT TECHNIQUES FOR THE SACRUM

(See Chapter 11.)

- Muscle energy: Forward torsion
- Muscle energy technique: Backward torsion
- High velocity, low amplitude technique: Anterior sacrum
- High velocity, low amplitude technique: Posterior sacrum

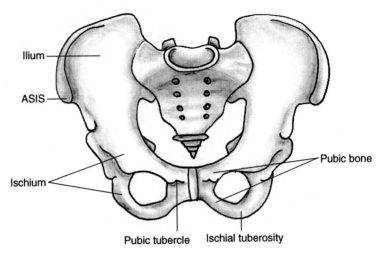

FIGURE 4-43. Pelvic anatomy—anterior view.

Pelvis

RELEVANT ANATOMY

(See Figures 4-43 and 4-44.)

- Formed from three fused bones: ilium, ischium, and pubic bone.
- Major bony landmarks are ASIS, PSIS, pubic tubercle, ischial tuberosity.
- In standing position, ASIS and pubic tubercle are in one frontal plane.

MOTION

- Rotation about the sacral inferior transverse sacral axis
- Also has some caliper motion, torsional motion, and superior/inferior translatory motion

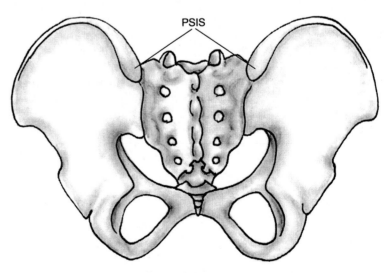

FIGURE 4-44. Posterior view of the pelvis.

DIAGNOSIS

- There are six main types of pelvic dysfunctions: anterior innominate, posterior innominate, superior innominate (up-slip), inferior innominate (down-slip), externally rotated (out-flared) innominate, internally rotated (in-flared) innominate.
- Innominate diagnosis involves five steps.
- **Step one:** Standing flexion test.
  - Tests iliosacral dysfunction. Tells you which side dysfunction is on, nothing more.
- **Step two:** Check position of ASIS.
- **Step three:** Check position of PSIS.
- **Step four:** Check pubic tubercles.
- **Step five:** Check ischial tuberosities.

ANTERIOR INNOMINATE

(See Figure 4-45.)

- Standing flexion test is positive on side of anterior innominate.
- Anterior superior iliac spine is inferior on affected side.
- Posterior superior iliac spine is superior on affected side.
- Pubic tubercle is inferior on affected side.
- Ischial tuberosity is superior on affected side.
- Can result in an apparent long leg on affected side.

POSTERIOR INNOMINATE

(See Figure 4-46.)

- Standing flexion test is positive on side of posterior innominate.
- Anterior superior iliac spine is superior on affected side.

Anterior innominate: Anterior landmarks are inferior while posterior landmarks are superior. Posterior innominate: Anterior landmarks are superior while posterior landmarks are inferior.

REGIONAL AND SYSTEMS-BASED ASSESSMENT

REGIONAL DIAGNOSIS

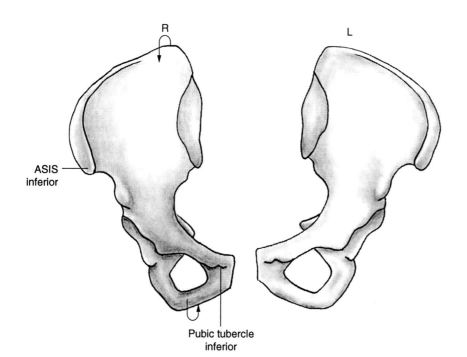

ASIS inferior

Pubic tubercle inferior

FIGURE 4-45. Anterior right innominate.

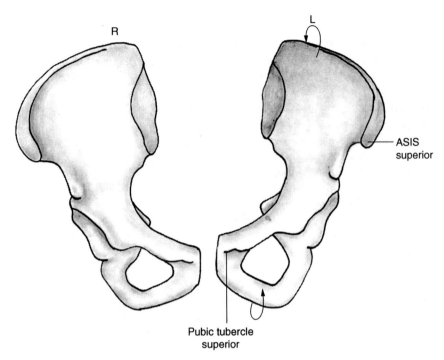

R   L

ASIS
superior

Pubic tubercle
superior

FIGURE 4-46. **Posterior left innominate.**

- Posterior superior iliac spine is inferior on affected side.
- Pubic tubercle is superior on affected side.
- Ischial tuberosity is inferior on affected side.
- Can result in an apparent short leg on affected side.

SUPERIOR INNOMINATE (A.K.A. UP-SLIP OR SUPERIOR SHEAR)

- Standing flexion test is positive on side of superior innominate.
- Anterior superior iliac spine is inferior on affected side.
- Posterior superior iliac spine is superior on affected side.
- Pubic tubercle is inferior on affected side.
- Ischial tuberosity is superior on affected side.
- Can result in an apparent long (a.k.a. inferior) leg on affected side.

INFERIOR INNOMINATE (A.K.A. DOWN-SLIP OR INFERIOR SHEAR)

- Standing flexion test is positive on side of inferior innominate.
- Anterior superior iliac spine is inferior on affected side.
- Posterior superior iliac spine is inferior on affected side.
- Pubic tubercle is inferior on affected side.
- Ischial tuberosity is inferior on affected side.
- Can result in an apparent long (a.k.a. inferior) leg on affected side.

EXTERNALLY ROTATED INNOMINATE (A.K.A. OUT-FLARE)

- Standing flexion test is positive on side of externally rotated innominate.
- Anterior superior iliac spine is lateral (relatively further from the midline) on affected side.
- Posterior superior iliac spine is medial (relatively closer to the midline) on affected side, resulting in a narrowed sacral sulcus on that side.

Superior innominate = everything superior on affected side! Inferior innominate = everything inferior on affected side!

Externally rotated innominate results in an externally rotated leg. Internally rotated innominate results in an internally rotated leg.

- Pubic tubercle is lateral on affected side.
- Ischial tuberosity is medial on affected side.
- Can result in an externally rotated leg on affected side.

INTERNALLY ROTATED INNOMINATE (A.K.A. IN-FLARE)

- Standing flexion test is positive on side of internally rotated innominate.
- Anterior superior iliac spine is medial on affected side.
- Posterior superior iliac spine is lateral on affected side, causing a widened sacral sulcus on that side.
- Pubic tubercle is medial on affected side.
- Ischial tuberosity is lateral on affected side.
- Can result in an internally rotated leg on affected side.

TREATMENT TECHNIQUES FOR THE PELVIS

- Muscle energy technique for anterior innominate
- Muscle energy technique for posterior innominate
- High velocity, low amplitude technique for innominate up-slip

▶ REVIEW QUESTIONS: SACRUM AND PELVIS DIAGNOSIS

Questions 1–2

A 42-year-old male presents to the clinic with low back pain. The patient states the pain started while he was shoveling snow the day before. The pain is focal, with no radiation to the extremities. There is acute tenderness over the right SI joint. L5 is flexed, sidebent, and rotated to the left. The left sacral sulcus is deep. The lumbosacral spring test is positive.

1. What is the diagnosis?
   A. Right on right forward torsion
   B. Left on left forward torsion
   C. Left on right forward torsion
   D. Left on right backward torsion
   E. Right on left backward torsion

2. To treat this dysfunction using ME, the patient should be positioned
   A. Supine
   B. Prone
   C. On the left side
   D. On the right side
   E. Seated

Questions 3–4

A 32-year-old female presents to the clinic with a 1-week history of low back pain. Seated flexion test is positive on the right. Lumbosacral spring test is negative. The right sulcus is deep.

3. You suspect a
   A. Left on left forward torsion
   B. Right on right forward torsion
   C. Left unilateral sacral flexion
   D. Right unilateral sacral extension
   E. Bilateral sacral flexion

4. You would expect L5 to be
   A. Flexed, sidebent left, rotated left
   B. Flexed, sidebent right, rotated right
   C. Neutral, rotated left, sidebent right
   D. Neutral, rotated right, sidebent left
   E. Extended, sidebent right, rotated left

Questions 5–6

A 45-year-old male presents to the clinic with low back pain ever since he moved the previous month. He describes focal pain over the left SI joint. The seated flexion test is positive on the left. There is tissue texture change over the left sacral sulcus, which is deeper than the right.

5. The sacrum is rotated _____ about a _____ oblique axis.
   A. Left, left
   B. Right, right
   C. Left, right
   D. Right, left
   E. All of the above

6. After treating his sacral dysfunction, you palpate his sacrum to determine the rate of his CRI. Cranial flexion and extension of the sacrum occurs about which axis?
   A. Superior transverse axis
   B. Middle transverse axis
   C. Inferior transverse axis
   D. Right oblique axis
   E. Left oblique axis

Questions 7–8

A 35-year-old male presents to the clinic with low back pain after cleaning his garage. The seated flexion test is positive on the right. The left sacral sulcus is deeper than the right. The right ILA is posterior.

7. You suspect
   A. Right unilateral flexion
   B. Right unilateral extension
   C. Right anterior sacrum
   D. Right posterior sacrum
   E. Bilateral sacral flexion

8. In order to treat this dysfunction using HVLA, the patient is positioned
   A. Prone, physician standing on patient's left
   B. Prone, physician standing on patient's right
   C. Supine, physician standing on patient's left
   D. Supine, physician standing on patient's right
   E. Laterally, on the side of the engaged oblique axis

Questions 9–10

A 63-year-old female presents to your office with severe right hip pain after walking to the grocery store yesterday. After a negative x-ray you decide to treat her using OMT. On examination, the standing flexion test is positive on the right. You notice her right ASIS is higher than her left, her right PSIS is higher than her left, and her right pubic tubercle is higher than her left.

9. You diagnose
   A. Right anterior innominate
   B. Right posterior innominate
   C. Right up-slip
   D. Right down-slip
   E. Right innominate out-flare

10. To treat this patient using HVLA, you would
    A. Extend and abduct the patient's leg
    B. Flex and internally rotate the patient's leg
    C. Extend and adduct the patient's leg
    D. Flex and abduct the patient's leg
    E. Extend and externally rotate the patient's leg

Questions 11–13

A 20-year-old female professional ballet dancer presents to the clinic with right-sided buttock pain after her partner dropped her during rehearsal 2 weeks ago. Her pain does not change with activity. However, she experiences some pain radiation down her right posterior thigh that stops at the knee when seated for an extended period of time. X-ray and magnetic resonance imaging (MRI) studies performed at an outside hospital were within normal limits. On physical examination, her lower extremity reflexes are +2/4 bilaterally, strength is +5/5 bilaterally, and gross sensation is intact. She has a positive right-seated flexion test and a deep sacral sulcus on the right.

11. With no further information, which of the following can you rule out?
    A. Left on left forward sacral torsion
    B. L5-S1 disk protrusion
    C. Right unilateral flexion
    D. Right anterior sacrum
    E. Left on right backward torsion
    F. Right on Left backward torsion
    G. Choices A, C, and F
    H. Both A and B
    I. Both B and F

12. In addition to what you have ruled out already, what other diagnosis can you rule out at this point and why?
    A. Right posterior sacrum because the seated flexion test is positive on the right
    B. Bilateral sacral flexion because you found a deep sacral sulcus on the right
    C. Bilateral sacral extension because the ILAs were posterior bilaterally

13. On further examination, you palpate tissue texture change in the right sacral sulcus at the upper pole of the SI joint. You also discover that the right ILA is posterior. What is your final diagnosis?
    A. Left on left forward sacral torsion
    B. Right on left backward torsion

C. Right unilateral sacral flexion

D. Right anterior sacrum

E. Left on right backward torsion

F. Right posterior sacrum

14. A 67-year-old man presents to the clinic with low back pain. Osteopathic structural examination reveals a positive seated flexion test on the right, a deep sulcus on the left, and a posterior ILA on the left. On palpation, tissue texture change is in the right sacral sulcus at the upper pole of the SI joint. What is the most likely SD that is causing the patient's lower back pain?

A. Left anterior sacrum

B. Left unilateral sacral flexion

C. Right on right forward torsion

D. Right unilateral sacral extension

E. Left posterior sacrum

15. A 55-year-old male limps into the clinic with severe low back pain. The patient claims that he can't stand up all the way since he "threw out his back." Orthopedic and neurological examinations are within normal limits. The seated flexion test and the sacral sulci are symmetrical. Sacral motion testing reveals the sacrum moving freely in flexion. Tissue texture changes in the sacral sulci are present bilaterally. Lumbosacral spring test is negative. What is the most likely diagnosis?

A. Left on right backward torsion

B. Bilateral sacral flexion

C. Right on left backward torsion

D. Right on right forward torsion

E. Bilateral sacral extension

> ▶ ANSWERS

1. **E**

This is a typical question you will see on boards. It contains more than enough information to make the diagnosis. First, we are given information about L5, which probably means the question is dealing with torsion. Second, L5 is flexed, sidebent, and rotated to the left. This tells us that we most likely have a backward torsion, the left oblique axis is engaged, and the sacrum is rotated to the right. The positive lumbosacral spring test helps confirm our suspicion. Finally, the left sulcus is deep (deeper than the right), which would give us a shallow sulcus on the right. If we know nothing else, we know L5 is sidebent left so the left oblique axis will be engaged. Looking at our answer choices, only B and E involve the left oblique axis. Of those two, only E is a backward torsion.

2. **C**

When treating either a forward or backward torsion using ME, the patient lays on the side of the involved oblique axis, in this case the left side.

3. **A**

This is a difficult question as it gives you very little information. However, only one answer choice fits with the information given. A right on right forward torsion would have a deep sulcus on the left. With a unilateral sacral flexion on the left, one would expect a deep sulcus on the left. In addition, the seated flexion test is positive on the right. With a unilateral sacral extension on the right, one would expect to see a deeper sulcus on the left. In addition, the lumbosacral spring test is negative, ruling out a sacral extension. The sulcus asymmetry and positive seated flexion test rule out a bilateral sacral dysfunction. Therefore, the only choice that potentially works is choice A, left on left forward torsion.

4. **D**

This question requires you to use the information in question three and work backward to come up with a diagnosis of L5. If we suspect a forward torsion, we know L5 will have neutral (Type I) mechanics, ruling out A, B, and E. If the sacrum is rotated left, we know L5 *always* rotates in the opposite direction of the sacrum, so the only answer choice that fits is D. Also, since the left oblique axis is engaged, we know L5 must be sidebent left, as the sidebending of L5 determines which axis is engaged.

5. **B**

This question gives us no information about L5 or the lumbosacral spring test; therefore, we suspect the question is not dealing with torsion. However, we're not being asked to diagnose a torsion or anterior/posterior sacrum. We're only being asked to diagnose sacral motion about an oblique axis. Looking at the answer choices, we know we're not dealing with a unilateral/bilateral sacral dysfunction because these only occur about the superior or middle transverse axes. Choice E can be ruled out immediately, as the sacrum does not simultaneously rotate about multiple oblique axes. Since it appears we're not dealing with the torsion model, choices C and D can be ruled out. In addition, we have tissue texture change over a deep sulcus. In a backward torsion, we would expect to have tissue texture change over a shallow sulcus. Since the seated flexion test, tissue texture changes, and sulcus depth all point to an anterior sacrum on the left (ie, right rotation about a right oblique axis), choice B becomes the best option. Even if we decided to call this a forward torsion (difficult to do since we have no information about L5), we would still come up with choice B. A left on left forward torsion would present with a deep sulcus on the right and the deep sulcus in this example is on the left.

6. **A**

This is a straightforward question asking about which axis cranial-sacral flexion and extension occurs. Anatomic flexion and extension occurs about the middle transverse axis. Innominate rotation occurs about the inferior transverse axis. Cranial-sacral flexion and extension does not occur about the oblique axes.

7. **D**

This is another question that gives us no information about the lumbar spine, so we suspect we're not dealing with a torsion question. In addition, looking at the answer choices, we know that torsion is not an option. The seated flexion test is positive on the right. This rules out choice E, as a bilateral sacral dysfunction would give us an equal-seated flexion test, equal sulcus depth, and equal ILA position. The remainder of the choices is on the right, so we cannot rule any of these out based on the seated flexion test alone. The left sulcus is deeper. This rules out choices A and C, which would have a deep sulcus on the right. Since the ILA is posterior on the opposite side of the deep sulcus, we know we are not dealing with a unilateral sacral dysfunction, leaving us with choice D.

8. C

The technique for treating a posterior sacrum using HVLA requires the patient to be supine. The physician stands on the opposite side of the dysfunction. Choice E would be correct for treating a forward or backward torsion using ME.

9. C

Since the standing flexion test is positive on the right, we know we have a right-sided problem. All the involved landmarks are higher on the right, giving us our diagnosis of an up-slip on the right.

10. B

To treat this using HVLA, we would use the leg pull technique. This involves slight flexion and internal rotation of the patient's leg.

11. I

Although this is a question addressing sacral SD, it is important to always rule out any orthopedic or neurological diagnoses in addition to any systemic diseases that can present as musculoskeletal complaints. This patient had unremarkable imaging studies and a normal neurological examination. The absence of these findings and the presence of palpable SDs allow you to comfortably rule out certain pathological diagnoses (for now). The positive right-seated flexion test *only* tells you that the problem is on the right side and nothing else. Knowing that the right sulcus is deeper than the left can allow you to begin narrowing your differential diagnosis. Choices A, C, D, and E would all cause a relative deep sulcus on the right with a positive right seated flexion test. A disc protrusion is unlikely considering the normal neurological examination along with an unremarkable MRI. A right on left backward torsion would create a positive seated flexion test on the right and a relative deep sulcus on the left.

12. B

All of the answer choices are unlikely but only choice B is unlikely for the right reason. A bilateral sacral flexion can be ruled out because you have found a deep sulcus on the right. The reason for this is when you have a bilateral sacral dysfunction, you won't have asymmetrical sulci; the sulci will either *both* be deep in a bilateral sacral flexion or *both* be shallow in a bilateral sacral extension. Since only one sulcus is deep, a bilateral flexion can comfortably be ruled out. Choice C, a bilateral sacral extension, will present with bilateral *anterior* ILAs; *however*, because you have not yet checked the ILAs, you cannot rule out this diagnosis based on the information given to this point. It is imperative that you look out for key words in the question stem that may be misleading. If you had already checked the ILAs, this answer choice would also be correct but the only information you have at this point is a positive seated flexion test and a deep sulcus on the right. Choice A is incorrect because a right-seated flexion test cannot rule out a right posterior sacrum. However, the deep right sulcus makes a right posterior sacrum unlikely.

13. C

Because the deep sulcus and the posterior ILA are on the same side, a right unilateral sacral flexion is the most likely diagnosis. When a posterior ILA is on the same side as the deep sulcus, then the sacrum is not engaged about an oblique axis. This makes all of the other answer choices unlikely, including the anterior/posterior sacral dysfunction. Also, if no information is given about L5, the dysfunction is less likely to be a forward or backward torsion.

14. D

This patient's presentation has a component of all the answer choices. In putting all the findings together, a right unilateral sacral extension, choice D, is the only choice that fits this clinical picture. The seated flexion test on the right tells you the problem is on the right. This eliminates choices A, B, and E. The tissue texture change confirms this. The deep sacral sulcus and the posterior ILA are on the same side; therefore, this is a unilateral dysfunction. This eliminates choice C.

15. B

The seated flexion test was symmetrical, which tells us that either the seated flexion test was negative (unlikely on a board question) or the test was positive bilaterally, strongly suggestive of a bilateral sacral dysfunction. The symmetrical sulci and tissue texture changes are also strongly suggestive of a bilateral sacral dysfunction, but neither of these findings is specific to a particular diagnosis. The negative lumbosacral spring test rules out bilateral sacral extension, leaving us with our diagnosis of a bilateral sacral flexion. Sacral motion testing revealing a sacrum that moves freely in flexion and resists extension, confirms the diagnosis.

> ► **EXTREMITY DIAGNOSIS**

Upper Extremity

RELEVANT ANATOMY

BONY

Scapula

- A triangular bone lying posterior to the rib cage, protected by strong muscular coverings.
- Winging of the scapula may occur with damage to the long thoracic nerve.

Clavicle

- A long bone that articulates medially with the manubrium of the sternum and laterally with the acromion of the scapula.
- Rarely, fragments from a clavicular fracture may damage the brachial vessels.

Humerus

- A long bone that articulates proximally with the glenoid fossa of the scapula and distally with the radius and ulna.
- A sharp blow to the posterior aspect of the medial epicondyle of the humerus may irritate the ulnar nerve.

Radius

- With pronation and supination, the radial head rotates around the radial notch of the ulna and the distal radius rotates on the head of the ulna.
- In the elderly, a fall on the hand produces a radial fracture 1 inch proximal to the wrist joint known as a Colles fracture.

Colles fracture: Radial fracture 1 inch proximal to the wrist joint.

Ulna

- The proximal portion of the ulna contains the olecranon. The trochlear fossa articulates with the humerus.
- Repeated trauma to the subcutaneous bursa overlying the olecranon causes an inflammation known as miner's elbow.

Carpal Bones

(See Figure 4-50.)

- The *carpus* is made of two rows: the proximal row and distal row.
- Proximal row consists of (from lateral to medial) the *scaphoid, lunate, triquetral, and pisiform.*
- Distal row consists of (from lateral to medial) the *trapezium, trapezoid, capitate, and hamate.*
- A fall on the palm with the hand abducted may cause a scaphoid fracture with resultant tenderness in the anatomic snuffbox and risk for potential avascular necrosis.

NERVOUS

- The brachial plexus (see Figure 4-47).
- Supplies the nerves of the upper extremity.
- Formed by nerve roots C5, C6, C7, C8, and T1.
- *Erb-Duchenne paralysis*: A brachial plexus injury which can occur during birth. A downward traction force can affect roots C5 and C6, causing the arm to hang limp at the patient's side with the forearm pronated and the palm facing backward.
- *Klumpke's paralysis*: Upward traction on the arm, during a forceful breech delivery, may tear roots C8 and T1, causing the hand to assume a clawed appearance.

SPECIFIC JOINTS

The Glenohumeral (Shoulder) Joint

(See Table 4-3.)

- Defined as the articulation between the head of the humerus and the glenoid fossa of the scapula.

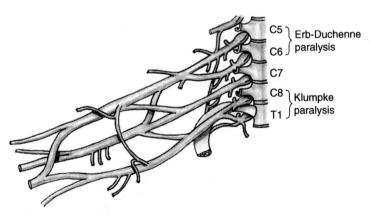

FIGURE 4-47. Brachial plexus.

ACTION	MUSCLE
Abduction	Supraspinatus, **deltoid (middle portion)**
Adduction	**Pectoralis major, latissimus dorsi,** subscapularis, infraspinatus, teres minor
Flexion	**Pectoralis major,** coraco-brachialis, **deltoid (anterior portion),** biceps brachii
Extension	Teres major, latissimus dorsi, **deltoid (posterior portion),** triceps brachii
Internal rotation	Pectoralis major, latissimus dorsi, deltoid, **subscapularis**
External rotation	**Infraspinatus,** teres minor, deltoid

Rotator Cuff

- The sheath of muscle tendons that aid in holding the head of the humerus in the glenoid cavity of the scapula during movements of the shoulder joint (Figure 4-48)
- Supraspinatus, infraspinatus, teres minor, subscapularis

DIAGNOSIS

Articular SD of the shoulder: Most often occurs at the sternoclavicular or acromioclavicular joints

- Dysfunction is characterized by pain at the involved joint and *restriction of motion* in one or more of the planes of joint motion.

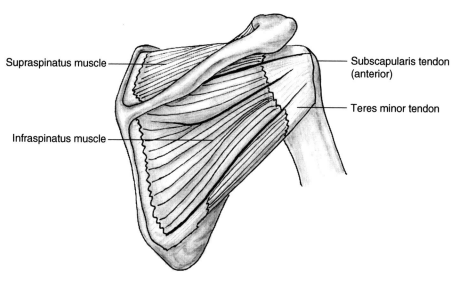

FIGURE 4-48. Rotator cuff.

- Restriction of motion in shoulder SD (compared to laxity in an orthopedic injury)
- Most common: Restriction in internal and external rotation
- Least common: Restriction in extension

SHOULDER PATHOLOGY

Shoulder Dislocation

- A traumatic repositioning of the humeral head outside the glenoid fossa of the scapula.
- The majority of shoulder dislocations occur anteriorly (in reference to infraglenoid tubercle). Traumatic forces in the anterior shoulder dislocation usually involve abduction and external rotation. This results in a humeral head that lies inferior to the glenoid fossa and anterior to the infraglenoid tubercle.

Rotator Cuff Tear

- Long-standing inflammation of the rotator cuff tendons caused by overuse, aging, a fall on an outstretched hand, or collision may lead to a disruption in one of the rotator cuff muscles.
- May also be caused by a mechanical impingement in an overhead position.
- The most common muscle involved in rotator cuff injury is the supraspinatus.

Frozen Shoulder (adhesive capsulitis)

- Constant limitation of the range of motion of the shoulder caused by scarring/adhesions in and around the shoulder joint.
- May be a consequence of rotator cuff disease and or associated with diabetes.

Impingement Syndrome

- Pain caused with elevation and internal rotation of the arm as the greater tuberosity of the humerus (with the supraspinatus riding on top) presses against the underside of the acromion.
- The Hawkins-Kennedy impingement test and Neer sign assess impingement syndrome by forward flexing the humerus with internal rotation (see Chapter 6).

TREATMENT TECHNIQUES FOR THE SHOULDER

(See Chapter 12.)

- Manipulation for the shoulder with ME
- Articulatory: Spencer seven-step technique
- Counterstrain: Coracoid tenderpoint counterstrain technique

THE ELBOW JOINT

- The true elbow joint is considered the ulnohumeral joint.
- The elbow is capable of 160° of flexion and 0° of extension around a transverse axis.
- Collateral ligaments stabilize the elbow laterally and medially. The musculature passing anterior and posterior to the elbow stabilize it anteroposteriorly.
- The carrying angle is defined as the angle formed by the intersection of two lines: one that passes down the long axis of the humerus, the other that starts at the proximal radial ulna joint and passes through the distal radial ulna joint (see Figure 4-49).

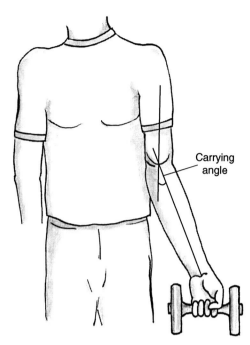

FIGURE 4-49. **Carrying angle.**

▪ Men typically have a normal carrying angle of 5°.
▪ Women typically have a carrying angle between 10° and 12°.

DIAGNOSIS

▪ Primary SD of the elbow is found in the ulnohumeral joint.
▪ Secondary SD is found at the radioulnar joint.
▪ During abduction of the ulna, the wrist is pushed into increased **adduction**.
▪ During adduction of the ulna, the wrist is pulled into **abduction**.
▪ An abduction SD of the ulna (adduction restriction) increases the carrying angle and causes the olecranon process to glide more freely medially. In an abducted ulna, the wrist will be adducted.
▪ An adduction SD of the ulna (abduction restriction) decreases the carrying angle and causes the olecranon process to glide more freely laterally. The wrist will also be abducted in this case.

In an abducted SD of the ulna, the wrist will be adducted.
In an adducted SD of the ulna, the wrist will be abducted.

ELBOW PATHOLOGY

Lateral Epicondylitis (tennis elbow)

▪ Often used as a blanket description for any soft tissue pain between the shoulder and wrist.
▪ Best defined as inflammation of the common extensor origin.
▪ Extensor carpi radialis brevis is the muscle most susceptible to irritation.
▪ Activities that combine repeated wrist extension with supination (tennis backhand, hammering, painting) are often responsible for the inflammation.

Medial Epicondylitis (golfer's elbow)

▪ Inflammation at the common flexor origin, affecting primarily the pronator teres muscle and the flexor carpi radialis muscle.
▪ Inflammation is provoked by activites involving powerful snapping of the wrist and pronation of the forearm.

Olecranon Bursitis

* Inflammation of the olecranon bursa located over the olecranon, subcutaneously.
* The bursa can become inflamed by leaning on the elbow for a prolonged period (a.k.a. student's elbow), or from a direct fall onto the point of the elbow.
* Impaired function of any joint of the arm produces compensatory changes in all other joints. If total functional demand overtaxes any one of the other joints, secondary SD is also produced in those joints.

TREATMENT TECHNIQUES FOR THE ELBOW

* High velocity, low amplitude: For anterior radial head and posterior radial head
* Muscle energy: Supination and pronation dysfunction
* Counterstrain: Lateral epicondyle tenderpoints

THE WRIST AND HAND

* The **true wrist** is defined as the ellipsoid radiocarpal joint formed by the distal end of the radius and the proximal carpal bones: scaphoid, lunate, and triquetral.
* The wrist has two axes of motion: the transverse axis and the AP axis.
* The hand and fingers consist of the distal carpal bones (trapezium, trapezoid, capitate, and hamate), five metacarpal bones, five proximal phalanges, four middle phalanges, and five distal phalanges.
* The thumb does not have a middle phalange.

DIAGNOSIS

SD of the Wrist

* Is related to the slight gliding motions of the carpal bones on the distal radius as the wrist is moved
* Is named according to the direction of freedom of motion (as with any SD)
* Is determined by comparing flexion to extension or abduction to adduction on both hands.
* Is usually caused by trauma if there is a flexion/extension SD. The trauma overcomes the ligamentous restrains and the opposing muscle pull

SD of the Hand

* Intercarpal SD usually occurs because of a fall on an outstretched hand.
* In the carpometacarpal joints (with the exception of the thumb), SD is primarily a dorsal glide with restriction of ventral glide.
* The metacarpophalangeal joints and interphalangeal joints may develop SD in the following:
  * Anteroposterior glide
  * Mediolateral glide
  * Internal/External rotational glide

WRIST AND HAND PATHOLOGY

Scaphoid Fracture

(See Figure 4-50.)

* A fracture of the scaphoid bone in the hand that occurs most commonly with a fall on an outstretched hand with the wrist fully extended.
* Fractures to the waist of the scaphoid bone may sever blood supply to the proximal portion of the bone leading to avascular necrosis.

The wrist flexes and extends around the transverse axis. It adducts and abducts around the AP axis.

Don't forget to rule out a scaphoid fracture, which can present as tenderness over the anatomical snuffbox.

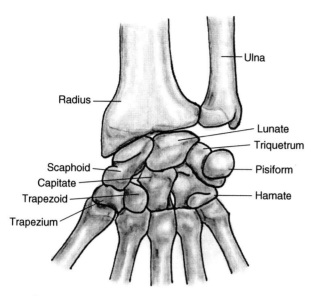

FIGURE 4-50. The wrist and carpal bones.

Carpal Tunnel Syndrome

- A compression neuropathy of the median nerve as it passes beneath the flexor retinaculum and into the carpal tunnel.
- Carpal tunnel syndrome is more common in women and typically occurs between the ages of 40 and 60.

De Quervain Syndrome

- An inflammation and thickening of the synovial lining of the common sheath of the abductor pollicis longus and extensor pollicis brevis tendons.
- Thickening occurs at the point where the tendon passes over the distal aspect of the radius.

TREATMENT TECHNIQUES FOR THE WRIST AND HAND

- Muscle energy: Wrist restriction in radial deviation
- Counterstrain: To treat wrist tenderpoints
- Metacarpal articulatory technique

Lower Extremity

RELEVANT ANATOMY

BONY

Femur

- Largest bone in the body.
- Consists of head, neck, shaft, and medial and lateral condyles.
- Fractures of the femoral neck (subcapital fractures) interrupt retinacular blood supply to the femoral head causing avascular necrosis.

Patella

- Sesamoid bone in the expansion of the quadriceps tendon.
- Continues from the apex of the bone as the ligamentum patellae.

■ Lateral dislocation of the patella is resisted by the prominent articular surface of the lateral condyle of the femur and the medial pull of the vastus medialis oblique (VMO) muscle.

Tibia

■ Long bone that expands proximally into the medial and lateral condyles.
■ Triangular shaft, which projects medially from the distal extremity of the bone as the medial malleolus.
■ Most common long bone to be fractured and to suffer compound injury.

The Q-Angle

(See Figure 4-51.)

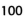

Increased Q-angle = genu vaLgus Decreased Q-angle = genu vaRum

■ Angle formed by the intersection of the longitudinal axis of the femur (a line drawn from the ASIS to the midpoint of the patella) and the longitudinal axis of the tibia (a line drawn through the midpoint of the patella and the tibial tubercle).
■ A normal Q-angle is 10° to 12°.
■ An abnormal Q-angle is >20°.
■ An increased Q-angle causes genu valgus (knock-knees).
■ A decreased Q-angle causes genu varum (bowleg).

Fibula

■ Serves as an origin for muscles, a part of the ankle joint, and a pulley for peroneus longus and brevis.
■ The bone consists of a head to which the fibularis longus and brevis attach, a neck, a shaft, and a lateral protuberance known as the lateral malleolus.
■ The fibula does not articulate with the femur at the knee joint.

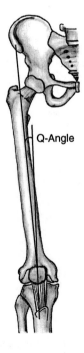

Q-Angle

FIGURE 4-51. The Q-angle.

Tarsal Bones

* Defined as the group of seven bones proximal to the metatarsal bones and phalanges.
* Seven tarsal bones are the talus, calcaneus, navicular, cuboid, and three cuneiforms.
* The bones of the foot also include 5 metatarsal bones and 14 phalanges.

NERVOUS

The Lumbar Plexus

(See Figure 4-52.)

* Originates from the anterior primary rami of L1 through L4.
* The principle branches of the lumbar plexus are the femoral nerve and obturator nerve.

The Sciatic Nerve

(See Figure 4-53.)

* Largest nerve in the body.
* Branches of the sciatic nerve supply the hamstring muscles (biceps femoris, semimembranosus, and semitendinosus) and the adductor magnus.
* *Sciatica* is defined as irritation of the sciatic nerve resulting in pain or tingling running down the leg and is often caused by a herniated lumbar disk.

    The sciatic nerve branches to form

* The tibial nerve—ends as the medial and lateral plantar nerves.
* The common peroneal nerve—divides to form the deep peroneal and superficial peroneal nerves.

SPECIFIC JOINTS

The Hip Joint

(See Table 4-4.)

* Largest joint in the body.
* Characterized as a ball and socket joint.
* The joint is deepened by a structure known as the acetabular labrum.

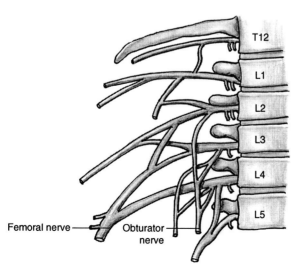

FIGURE 4-52. The lumbar plexus.

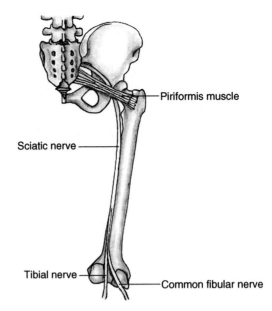

FIGURE 4-53. Sciatic nerve.

DIAGNOSIS

Hip SD

- Characterized by a relative decrease in typical range of motion.
- Gait may appear abnormal.
- Muscles surrounding the hip joint demonstrate tenderpoints at the muscle origin and insertion.

TABLE 4-4. Motion at the Hip Joint (bolded muscles represent the primary muscles involved in the action)

ACTION	MUSCLE
Abduction	**Gluteus medius, gluteus minimus,** tensor fasciae latae, sartorius
Adduction	**Adductor longus, brevis and magnus, gracilis,** pectineus
Flexion	**Iliacus and psoas,** rectus femoris, sartorius, pectineus, and tensor fasciae latae
Extension	**Gluteus maximus, hamstrings**
Lateral rotation	**Gluteus maximus,** the obturators, gemelli, sartorius, quadratus femoris, and piriformis
Medial rotation	Tensor fasciae latae and anterior fibers of **gluteus medius and minimus**

Psoasitis SD

- Patient typically presents with flexion at the waist and slightly bent to the side of the aggravated psoas.
- Leg extension is restricted.

(See Table 4-2 for more on psoas SD.)

Gluteus Maximus SD

- Somatic dysfunction of gluteus maximus leads to restriction of hip flexion and internal rotation.
- Dysfunction of gluteus medius and minimus may decrease leg abduction.

Piriformis SD

- Restriction of leg internal rotation.
- Possible numbness and tingling in the back of the leg, mimicking sciatica.

HIP PATHOLOGY

Legg-Calvé-Perthes Disease

- Avascular necrosis of the femoral head causing the bony nucleus of the epiphysis to become necrosed
- May be caused by joint effusion at the hip following trauma

Slipped Capital Femoral Epiphysis

(See Figure 4-54.)

- A posterior and inferior slippage of the proximal femoral epiphysis on the femoral neck occurring through the physeal plate during the early adolescent growth spurt
- The most common hip disorder in adolescents

Clicking Hip Syndrome

- Snapping in the hip that can be painful or not painful.
- Common in dancers and young athletes.
- External hip click is usually caused by the movement of the gluteus maximus tendon or ilio-tibial band clicking over the greater trochanter.
- Internal hip click caused by movement of the iliopsoas over its bursa.

LEG radiculopathies are caused by spasm of the piriformis muscle, which lies in close proximity to the sciatic nerve.

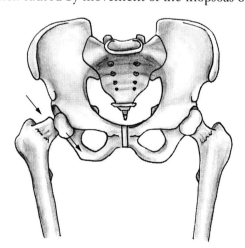

FIGURE 4-54. Slipped capital femoral epiphysis.

TREATMENT TECHNIQUES FOR THE HIP

- Muscle energy: Psoas muscle spasm
- Counterstrain: Piriformis

THE KNEE JOINT

- Most complicated articulation in the body.
- Consists of a medial and lateral femoral-tibial articulation and a patellofemoral articulation, all within one joint capsule.
- One of the few joints with menisci.
- The quadriceps muscles, the quadriceps tendon, and the patellar tendon maintain the stability of the patellofemoral joint.

DIAGNOSIS

Adduction Dysfunction—Tibia on Femur

- A condition of **varus** stress of the tibia on the femur

Abduction Dysfunction—Tibia on Femur

- A condition of **valgus** stress of the tibia on the femur

Anterior-Posterior Glide Dysfunction

- The tibia is restricted in anterior or posterior glide. The initial patient complaints are restrictions of flexion or extension movements.

KNEE PATHOLOGY

Meniscal Tears

- Tear in the shock-absorbing fibrocartilage of the knee.
- Most common reason for arthroscopy of the knee.
- Most frequently occurs in the medial meniscus, which is securely attached around the entire periphery of the joint capsule.

Anterior Cruciate Ligament Tear

- Tear of the ligament that prevents anterior translation of the tibia on the femur or posterior translation of the femur on a fixed tibia.
- Most common knee ligament injury.

Posterior Cruciate Ligament Tear

- Tear of the ligament that prevents posterior translation of the tibia on the femur (or anterior translation of femur on fixed tibia).
- Much less common than a tear to the anterior cruciate ligament (ACL).

Patellofemoral Pain Syndrome

- Pain to the undersurface of the patella, attributed to cartilage damage on the posterior surface of the patella.
- Damage results from the patella not riding within the femoral groove.
- Poor tracking of the patella within the femoral groove may be attributed to VMO weakness and a positive "J sign" may be present on physical examination (Figure 4-55).

TREATMENT TECHNIQUES FOR THE KNEE

- High velocity, low amplitude: Anterior fibular head dysfunction
- Counterstrain: Patellar tenderpoint

A blow to the medial knee joint or a twisting motion that produces lateral ligamentous sprain may result in an adduction dysfunction.

A blow to the lateral knee joint or a twisting motion that produces medial ligamentous sprain may result in an abduction dysfunction.

The terrible triad = rupture of the ACL, medial collateral ligament, and the medial meniscus from a blow to the lateral knee.

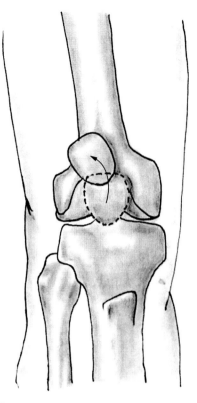

FIGURE 4-55. *"J sign".*

THE ANKLE AND FOOT

- The distal end of the tibia, the medial malleoli, and the lateral malleoli make up the crural arch (also known as the ankle mortise), which snuggly holds the talus.
- The joint capsule, the deltoid ligaments, the anterior talofibular ligament (ATFL), the posterior talofibular ligament (PTFL), the anterior and posterior tibiofibular ligaments, and the calcaneofibular ligament (CFL) connect the above bones.
- The ankle joint is most stable in dorsiflexion (because of the anterior aspect of the talus wedging between the malleoli).

DIAGNOSIS

- Somatic dysfunction of the ankle often follows immobilization and is characterized by restriction of motion.
- Talar dysfunction at the tibiotalar joint is a common lower extremity dysfunction. The talus is often restricted in dorsiflexion.
- Restriction at the tarsal and metatarsal joints is most effectively diagnosed with dorsal and plantar motion testing.

ANKLE AND FOOT PATHOLOGY

Ankle Inversion Sprain

- Sprain or tear of the lateral ligamentous structures surrounding the ankle joint.
- Anterior talofibular ligament is most commonly affected (ATFL > CFL > PTFL).
- Can also cause lateral malleolus SD as well as a "dropped" cuboid.

Distal tibiofibular dysfunction often resolves with treatment of the proximal tibiofibular articulation.

105

Medial Ankle Sprain

- Sprain or tear of the deltoid complex induced by pathological abduction and pronation of the foot.

Plantar Fasciitis

- Chronic irritation of the plantar fascia, usually a result of biomechanical imbalances.

TREATMENT TECHNIQUES FOR THE ANKLE AND FOOT

- Counterstrain: Medial ankle tenderpoint
- High velocity, low amplitude: Cuboid and navicular SD
- Articulation: Metatarsal heads

> ▶ **REVIEW QUESTIONS: EXTREMITY DIAGNOSIS**

1. Upon motion testing the elbow joint, you notice that the olecranon process glides more freely medially. Consequently, you notice that the wrist moves further into
   A. Pronation
   B. Supination
   C. Adduction
   D. Abduction
   E. Flexion

2. Upon physical examination of a 30-year-old female, you note that her carrying angle measures approximately 15°. The normal carrying angle for a woman is between
   A. 10° and 12°
   B. 5° and 10°
   C. 15° and 18°
   D. 8° and 10°
   E. 18° and 20°

3. A 40-year-old carpenter enters the clinic complaining of tenderness on the lateral aspect of his forearm, just distal to the elbow. He states that the pain is particularly severe when he uses a screwdriver, and that ibuprofen reduces his discomfort minimally. You suspect that his pain results from repetitive overuse and you tell him that his condition is most commonly known as
   A. Miner's elbow
   B. Nursemaids' elbow
   C. Olecranon bursitis
   D. Tennis elbow
   E. Washwoman's elbow

4. A 35-year-old female presents to the clinic with low back pain and muscle spasm. You note that she is flexed at the waist but also slightly bent to the right side. She refuses to lie prone on the table and, instead, prefers to lie on her back with her knees pulled to her chest. What is the most likely etiology of her pain?
   A. Right quadratus lumborum spasm
   B. Right piriformis spasm

C. Left piriformis spasm

D. L4 to L5 disk herniation

E. Right psoas spasm

5. A 25-year-old male presents to the clinic after "twisting" his knee during a basketball game. He states that he has experienced several episodes of sharp, shooting pain on the medial aspect of his knee since the accident and that he hears an occasional "click" when he's walking. The patient states that the day before, while walking down the stairs, his knee "gave out." The most likely structure injured is the

A. ACL

B. Posterior cruciate ligament

C. Medial meniscus

D. Lateral meniscus

E. Patella

6. A 15-year-old girl presents to the emergency room (ER) after hurting her ankle during a soccer game. She says that she stepped on an opponent's foot, inverting her foot. The ankle demonstrates inflammation over the lateral malleolus and slight discoloration. The x-ray is negative. You suspect an inversion sprain and assess for which SD?

A. Dropped cuboid

B. Dropped navicular

C. Anterior fibular head

D. Posterior fibular head

E. Tibial torsion

▶ ANSWERS

1. **C**

During abduction of the ulna, the wrist is pushed into increased adduction. During adduction of the ulna, the wrist is pulled into abduction. An abduction SD increases *abduction* of the ulna and further wrist *adduction*.

2. **A**

The normal carrying angle for women is between 10° and 12°.

3. **D**

Lateral epicondylitis is most commonly known as tennis elbow.

4. **E**

The patient most likely suffers from a right psoas spasm. Patients with acute psoas spasm typically present with flexion at the waist and are slightly bent to the side of the dysfunctional psoas.

5. **C**

The patient in this question presents with signs and symptoms consistent with a meniscal tear. As the symptoms are on the medial side, we would suspect the medial meniscus as the probable structure injured.

6. **A**

A dropped cuboid commonly accompanies an inversion sprain.

CHAPTER 5

Osteopathic Principles and Considerations of Clinical Medicine: A Systems-Based Approach

Often osteopathic manipulative medicine (OMM) questions on the boards are part of a much bigger clinical scenario. They can catch you off guard if you don't keep the basic principles in the back of your head while taking the test. One of the more high-yield areas of OMM and the systemic systems is the principle of the normalization of the autonomic nervous system (ANS). Understanding the sympathetic and parasympathetic effects on each system is imperative. In addition, the viscerosomatic reflex(es) (VSR) must be reviewed. Remember, the autonomic innervation of the organs does not always correlate with the VSR. They are extremely similar, but keep the differences in mind when differentiating questions regarding the ANS and questions regarding the VSR. Another high-yield topic tends to focus on appropriate techniques for specific pathology. This section discusses OMM within each system of the body. The relevant anatomy, VSR, osteopathic considerations, and treatment guidelines will all be reviewed. This is *not* intended to be a medicine review but, rather, an organized approach to incorporating OMM into your clinical problem-solving skills.

▶ HEAD, EARS, EYES, NOSE, THROAT

Introduction

Head, ears, eyes, nose, throat (HEENT) complaints are some of the most common complaints in the primary care setting ranging from headaches (HAs) and sinusitis to ear infections and sore throats. As usual, OMM questions on the boards will focus on VSR as well as appropriate techniques. A few key points to remember include normalizing the sympathetics to the head (T1-T4); when in doubt, pick a lymphatic technique for treatment, if possible, and focus on techniques that will indirectly affect the head (ie, cervical and thoracic techniques). Rarely will you see something specific about facial techniques.

Relevant Anatomy

- Internal carotid arteries pass through the carotid canal in the petrous portion of the temporal bone.
- Vertebral arteries enter through the foramen magnum.
- Internal jugular veins pass through the jugular foramina.
- Deep cervical lymph nodes are located along the internal jugular veins.
- Cranial nerve (CN) V—trigeminal nerve.
- V1 (ophthalmic division)—passes through the cavernous sinus and enters the orbit through the superior orbital fissure (treatment at the superior orbital foramina affects this division).
- V2 (maxillary division)—passes through the foramen rotundum of the sphenoid and enters the orbit through the inferior orbital fissure (treatment at the inferior orbital foramina affects this division).
- V3 (mandibular division)—passes through the foramen ovale of the sphenoid (treatment at the mental foramina affects this division).
- Cranial nerve VII—facial nerve.
- Enters the internal acoustic meatus of the temporal bone and exits at the stylomastoid foramina of the temporal bone.
- Cranial nerve VIII—vestibulocochlear nerve.
- Enters the internal acoustic meatus with CN VII.

Generalized VSR for HEENT

SYMPATHETICS—T1 TO T4

- Increased sympathetic tone leads to photophobia, tinnitus, unsteady gait.
- Prolonged sympathetic tone leads to thick and sticky nasal and pharyngeal secretions.

PARASYMPATHETICS—CN V, OCCIPUT, C1 AND C2

- Increased parasympathetic activity leads to excessive tear production and profuse, thin nasopharyngeal and sinus secretions.

  (For a more specific listing, please refer to Viscerosomatic Reflexes, Chapter 6.)

Osteopathic Considerations and Treatment Guidelines for HEENT Pathology

DYSFUNCTION AFFECTING RELEVANT ANATOMIC STRUCTURES

ARTERIAL

- Cranial dysfunction of temporals, occiput, or sphenoid can affect the internal carotid arteries; signs and symptoms include weakness and altered sensation on the contralateral side.
- Cervical dysfunction from C2 to C6 can affect the vertebral arteries; signs and symptoms include dizziness and visual abnormalities.

VENOUS

- Cranial dysfunction of the temporals, specifically occipitomastoid compression, can affect the venous drainage (internal jugular veins); signs and symptoms include head congestion.

LYMPHATICS

- Somatic dysfunction of the upper thoracic spine, upper ribs, and clavicle can affect the lymphatic system; signs and symptoms include head congestion which may be more specifically because of decreased drainage through the thoracic inlet.

CRANIAL NERVES

- Cranial dysfunction of the temporals can affect V1 leading to problems in the distribution of V1.
- Cranial dysfunction of the temporals, sphenoid, maxillae, and mandible can affect V2 leading to problems in the distribution of V2, and more specifically, Tic douloureux (intense paroxysmal neuralgia along the trigeminal nerve).
- Dysfunction of the temporal mandibular joint (TMJ) and other problems with the mouth and teeth (poorly fitted dentures) can affect V3 leading to HAs.
- Dysfunction of the sphenoid, occiput, temporals, and cervical fascia can affect CN VII; signs and symptoms include eyelid spasms and Bell palsy (facial nerve paralysis).
- Dysfunction of the sphenoid, occiput, and temporals can affect CN VIII; signs and symptoms include hearing impairment and vertigo.

OTHER COMMON HEENT PATHOLOGY

Attention: Causes are defined by osteopathic parameters.

SINUSITIS

- Cause: Cranial dysfunction preventing adequate drainage of the paranasal sinuses.
- Treatment guidelines: Remove the dysfunctional cranial motion patterns.
- Frontal sinuses: Use frontal lift.
- Ethmoid sinus: Use frontal lift, vomer pump, facial articulatory techniques.
- Sphenoid sinuses: Correct cranial strain patterns.
- Maxillary sinuses: Use frontal lift or facial articulatory techniques.

All treatment for the mentioned manifestations of common HEENT pathology should focus on treating the cranial dysfunctions that are causing the problem.

OTITIS MEDIA

- Cause: Internal rotation of the temporal bone may result in partial or complete closure of the eustachian tube leading to impaired drainage.
- Treatment guidelines: The Galbreath technique.

VERTIGO

- Cause: Temporal bone dysfunction (internal or external rotation) can alter the normal position and function of the vestibular apparatus.
- Treatment guidelines: Cranial techniques affecting the temporal bone.

COMMON COLD

- Cause: No specific osteopathic consideration.
- Treatment guidelines: Support the body and establish an environment for healing to occur.
- Improve arterial supply to, and venous/lymphatic drainage away from, the head and neck (treat the neck, upper back, and ribs; use lymphatic techniques).
- Facilitate breathing (treat the diaphragm and ribs).

HEADACHES

Tension Type HAs

- Cause: Can be caused by somatic dysfunction (SD) in the upper thoracics, cervical region, and cranium; also consider poor posture or poor work setup.
- Treatment guidelines:
  - Address postural issues with exercises.
  - Address work environment issues (ie, raising computer screen, changing chair height).
  - Use high velocity, low amplitude (HVLA), muscle energy (ME), soft tissue (ST), counterstrain (CS), myofascial release (MFR) where appropriate.
  - Specifically, focus on tight scalenes, suboccipital tension, and occipital-atlantal joint and type II upper thoracic SDs.
  - Migraine HAs
- Cause: Can be triggered by stress, odors, foods, alcohol, and menstruation
- Treatment guidelines
  - Check patients vision as eye strain can lead to migraines.
  - Reduce tension in the body via treatment to the upper thoracics, head, and neck.

■ Exercise and stretching programs target tension reduction throughout the body and release endorphins, thus providing natural prophylactic treatment.

■ Treatment is best applied between HAs, but can be beneficial during the migraine episode by utilizing cranial techniques focusing on the temporals, frontals, and occiput bones.

Cluster HAs

■ Cause and treatments are similar to that of migraine HAs.
■ Treatment may need to be more frequent to break cycle.

▶ REVIEW QUESTIONS: HEENT

1. A 35-year-old male presents to his primary care physician with complaints of vision abnormalities and dizziness for the past 2 weeks. The patient's physical examination was unremarkable except for tissue texture change and motion restriction in the area of C5 and throughout the thoracic spine. The patient's lesion at C5 may contribute to his dizziness and vision changes by affecting the
   A. Vagal nerve
   B. Brachial plexus
   C. Anterior scalenes
   D. Vertebral artery
   E. Spinal cord

2. A 44-year-old female presents to her primary care physician complaining of a noticeable droop on the right side of her face and inability to close her right eye. She states that she has been drooling and having trouble speaking. The CN responsible for the patient's symptoms is CN
   A. VI
   B. VIII
   C. VII
   D. VIII
   E. IX

3. (Referring to the above patient.) The physician suspects a cranial dysfunction is responsible for the patient's symptoms. Dysfunction of which cranial bone will most likely cause the above patient's symptoms?
   A. The parietal bone
   B. The temporal bone
   C. The frontal bone
   D. The lacrimal bone
   E. The maxilla

4. A 4-year-old child presents to his primary care physician with recurrent otitis media of his right ear. Upon evaluating the child's cranial motion, the physician notices that the child's right temporal bone is
   A. Externally rotated
   B. Flexed
   C. Extended
   D. Torsioned
   E. Internally rotated

114

5. A 55-year-old male presents to the emergency room (ER) with a headache that he describes as "stabbing" and "excruciating" behind his right eye. The pain began 2 hours ago. The patient states that he has had similar HAs in the past and that they usually go away after 3 hours. The most likely diagnosis is
   A. Cluster headache
   B. Meningioma
   C. Migraine headache
   D. Tension headache
   E. Epidural hematoma

1. **D**

The vertebral arteries pass through the transverse foramen in the cervical spine. Somatic dysfunction in the cervical spine, particularly levels C2 to C6, may affect the vertebral arteries causing dizziness and vision changes.

2. **C**

This case is describing a classic Bell palsy, which is a condition characterized by facial paralysis and associated with CN VII.

3. **B**

Bell palsy is a condition associated with the facial nerve, CN VII. Cranial dysfunction associated with Bell palsy can occur with dysfunction of the temporals, sphenoid, or occiput.

4. **E**

Internal rotation on the temporal bone may result in partial or complete closure of the eustachian tube, inhibiting drainage of the middle ear, and establishing an appropriate medium for otitis media.

5. **E**

Cluster HAs are characterized by stabbing, retro-orbital pain that lasts between 15 minutes and 3 hours. Attacks may be seasonal and followed by months of remission.

► CARDIOLOGY

Introduction

Many cardiac conditions are not caused by dysfunction of the musculoskeletal system but may result in dysfunction of the somatic system. The acute cardiac conditions obviously need to be dealt with medically first, and osteopathic manipulative techniques (OMT) may not be a first line of treatment. However, most conditions will be associated with particular VSR and many conditions will respond to OMT in the later stages or chronic disease states. Treatment guidelines will be given when appropriate.

Relevant Anatomy

- Sympathetic innervation.
  - T1 to T4.
  - Accelerates the heart.

- Parasympathetic innervation.
  - Cranial nerve X (vagus).
  - Decelerates the heart.
- Both divisions of the ANS come together at the cardiac plexus.

Generalized VSR for the Cardiac System

- Sympathetics—T1 to T5 (left > right)
- Parasympathetics—C0, C1, mainly C2 (vagus)

  (For a more specific listing, please refer to Viscerosomatic Reflexes, Chapter 6.)

Osteopathic Considerations and Treatment Guidelines for Cardiac Pathology

MYOCARDIAL INFARCTION

- Acute phase
  - Stabilize the patient. Now is not the time to work on your Kirksville crunch.
  - Use **VSR** to help with diagnosis.
  - Changes may be found over the rib angles and at T2 on the left.
  - Any direct OMT and lymphatic pump techniques are contraindicated.
- Post-myocardial infarction (MI) treatment guidelines:
  - Restore motion to the thoracic spine (ST, deep articulation [DA]).
  - Normalize autonomics (treat occipitoatlantal [OA] and C2 to restore parasympathetic tone).
  - Consider diaphragm release and rib raising techniques.
  - Apply thoracic inlet and fascial release techniques.

CONGESTIVE HEART FAILURE

- Musculoskeletal manifestations:
  - Swelling in the lower extremities (may complain of recent weight gain).
  - Dyspnea on exertion (DOE) or difficulty breathing at rest.
  - Somatic dysfunction—tissue texture change in the upper thoracics (VSR) and in the upper cervical (parasympathetic innervation to the heart, specifically C2, vagus).
- Treatment guidelines: Improve venous and lymphatic return (be careful not to overtax the cardiovascular [CV] system during an acute attack),
  - Treat the respiratory diaphragm (indirect balancing).
  - Treat the pelvic diaphragm.
  - Treat the thoracic cage and outlet (MFR, ST, DA, ME).
  - Treat the VSR (T1-T5 for the head, T9-L1 for the kidneys).

HYPERTENSION

- Treatment guidelines:
  - Lower thoracic treatment to affect facilitation to the adrenals/renals.
  - Cervical/upper thoracic treatment to affect facilitation to the heart.
  - Occipitoatlantal and C2 treatment to affect parasympathetic innervation to the heart.
  - Rib treatment to affect the sympathetic chain.

1. A 66-year-old male presents to the ER with "crushing" pain beneath his sternum that radiates to his jaw and left arm. He is diaphoretic and appears ashen. You suspect an MI. Palpation may reveal tissue texture change
   A. In the thoracic spine, T2, left
   B. In the thoracic spine, T6, right
   C. In the cervical spine, C1, right
   D. In the thoracic spine, T12, left
   E. Over the tenth rib, right

2. The anterior Chapman reflex points (CRP) for an MI appears
   A. Between the second and third transverse processes
   B. At the fifth intercostal space
   C. Along the midline of the sternum
   D. At the second intercostal space, next to the sternum
   E. Immediately below the xyphoid process

3. A physician suspects kidney involvement in a patient's sudden-onset hypertension. To help confirm his suspicions, he may look for a CRP
   A. At a distance of 2.5 inch above the umbilicus, on either side of the median line
   B. One in above the umbilicus, on either side of the median line
   C. On either side of the lumbar spinous processes
   D. At the angle of the twelfth rib
   E. Immediately below the costal margin, anteriorly

Questions 4–5

A patient presents to the ER with a HA, sweating, palpitations, chest pain, and abdominal pain. On physical examination, you note a hand tremor. His blood pressure is 180/90 mm Hg. The abdominal computerized tomography (CT) scan shows a small adrenal mass that you suspect to be a pheochromocytoma.

4. When palpating for CRPs, you expect to find one
   A. At a distance of 2.5 inch above, and 1 inch on either side of the umbilicus
   B. One in above the umbilicus, on either side of the median line
   C. On either side of the lumbar spinous processes
   D. At the angle of the twelfth rib
   E. Immediately below the costal margin, anteriorly

5. In addition to medical treatment for this patient, you decide to use OMT to help normalize sympathetic tone. Which technique would be most appropriate?
   A. Cervical ST
   B. Muscle energy to the atlas
   C. Rib raising
   D. Myofascial release of the diaphragm
   E. Pedal pump

1. A

Viscerosomatic change related to MI generally appears in the thoracic spine, in the areas of T1 to T5. Findings are more commonly on the left than on the right.

2. D

The anterior CRPs, generally associated with an MI, are located at the second intercostal space, next to the sternum.

3. B

The CRPs for the kidney appear on either side of the median line, 1 inch above the umbilicus.

4. A

Chapman reflex points, associated with the adrenal glands, appear 2.5 inch above and 1 inch on either side of the umbilicus.

5. C

While each of these techniques may be of benefit, rib raising acts on the sympathetic chain aiding in normalization of sympathetic tone.

▶ **PULMONOLOGY**

Introduction

Diseases of the respiratory system are commonly associated with SD. Asthma, bronchitis, and pneumonia are only three examples. Although COMLEX questions focus primarily on respiratory VSR, some questions highlight treatment techniques for the pulmonary patient. Many of the techniques increase mobility of the related somatic components and can be used on patients with a variety of pulmonary disease processes.

Relevant Anatomy

THORACIC CAGE

- Bony components: Cervical and thoracic vertebrae, ribs, sternum, manubrium
- Muscles: Paraspinals, intercostals, diaphragm (some people use accessory muscles for respiration, ie, SCM and scalenes)
- Joints: Costovertebral, costotransverse, costochondral, costosternal

Thoracic Inlet—Anatomical

- T1 vertebrae
- The superior end of the manubrium
- The first ribs and their costal cartilages

Thoracic Inlet—Functional

- T1 to T4 vertebrae
- The manubrium of the sternum
- Ribs 1 and 2, plus costicartilages

Generalized VSR for the Pulmonary System

- Sympathetics—T1 to T4, bilateral
- Parasympathetics—C0, C1, C2 (vagus), C3 to C5 (phrenic)

(For a more specific listing, please refer to Viscerosomatic Reflexes, Chapter 6.)

Osteopathic Considerations and Treatment Guidelines for Pulmonary Pathology

DYSFUNCTION AFFECTING RELEVANT ANATOMIC STRUCTURES

THORACIC OUTLET SYNDROME

- An entrapment syndrome of various nerves, arteries, and lymphatics, such as the brachial plexus trunks and subclabian vessels which supply the arms.
- Entrapment (primarily of the brachial plexus) occurs over the slope of the first rib, between the anterior and middle scalene muscles, or beneath the pectoralis minor muscle.
- Regular employment of accessory muscles of respiration may predispose a patient to thoracic outlet syndrome.

A positive Adson test can indicate thoracic outlet syndrome. See page 162 for a description of the Adson test.

CERVICAL VERTEBRAE DYSFUNCTION

- C0, C1, mainly C2 (vagus)—provide parasympathetic innervation to the lower respiratory tract.
  - Dysfunction may lead to bronchospasm.
- C3 to C5—phrenic nerve originates here.
  - Dysfunction may lead to restrictions within the diaphragm.

OTHER COMMON PULMONARY PATHOLOGY

COUGH

- Associated with diseases of the respiratory system as well as diseases of the cardiovascular and gastrointestinal (GI) systems.
- Related SD:
  - Upper thoracic segmental dysfunction—secondary to VSR or the added mechanical stresses of coughing
    - Dysfunctions are primarily Type II in nature—sidebent and rotated to the same side with a flexion/extension component.
  - Rib dysfunction
    - Positional—posterior ribs are most commonly found.
    - Functional—both inhaled or exhaled ribs can be found on structural examination.
  - Muscular dysfunction—spasm of the intercostals, paraspinals, and scalenes
- Treatment guidelines:
  - Treat the upper thoracics—HVLA, ME, CS
  - Treat the ribs—HVLA, ME, CS
  - Treat the VSR (upper cervicals)—indirect balancing of C2, FPR

ASTHMA

- A reversible obstructive airway disease characterized by airway inflammation and hypersensitivity
- Treatment reminders
  - Always treat the acute patient with the appropriate medical means first.
  - Treatment guidelines for the chronic asthmatic (between attacks) focus on the VSR.

BRONCHITIS AND PNEUMONIA

- Leads to a buildup of mucus within the bronchioles
- Result in difficulty with inhalation and exhalation
- Treatment regimen
  - Improve lymphatic and venous flow—lymphatic pump, MFR of thoracic outlet.
  - Decrease bronchial secretions—rib raising.
  - Decrease the work load of breathing—indirect balancing of the diaphragm.
  - Treat the upper thoracics, ribs, and cervicals (VSR)—HVLA, ME, CS, FPR.

CHRONIC OBSTRUCTIVE PULMONARY DISEASE

- Associated with musculoskeletal changes—barrel chest, hypertrophy of accessory muscles of respiration (sternocleidomastoid [SCM], scalenes), restriction of rib motion, increased kyphosis of thoracic spine, restriction of the diaphragm
- Treatment guidelines
  - Mobilize the thoracic spine and ribs—ST, DA, ME, CS, FPR.
  - Mobilize the diaphragm—indirect balancing.
  - Improve lymphatic and venous flow—lymphatic pump, MFR of thoracic outlet.
  - Treat the VSR.

► **REVIEW QUESTIONS: PULMONARY**

Questions 1–5

An 88-year-old male presents to the clinic for evaluation of long-standing emphysema. In addition to standard therapy for this condition, you have been treating him using OMT.

1. Which of the following would not be an appropriate treatment to use on this patient?
   A. Indirect treatment of the atlas
   B. Thoracic outlet MFR
   C. Diaphragm release
   D. Thoracic lymphatic pump
   E. Pedal lymphatic pump

2. The patient states he has been coughing recently. What SD findings might you expect to find on this patient?
   A. Hypertonic scalenes
   B. Flexed upper thoracic lesions
   C. Exhaled rib dysfunction
   D. Restricted diaphragm
   E. All of the above

3. Which region of the spine would you focus on to normalize parasympathetic tone to the diaphragm in this patient?
   A. C2
   B. T2
   C. T12
   D. L2
   E. Sacrum

4. The diaphragm is innervated by which cervical roots?
   A. C1 to C3
   B. C2 to C4
   C. C3 to C5
   D. C4 to C6
   E. C5 to C7

5. The patient thanks you for your treatment and wants to know if there is anything he can do by himself while at home to help his SD. Which would be the most appropriate treatment to recommend?
   A. CV4
   B. Scalene ME
   C. Myofascial release of the diaphragm
   D. Thoracic HVLA
   E. Muscle energy for a forward torsion

Questions 6–7

A patient comes into your clinic complaining of diffuse right arm pain. He is a window cleaner and his job has become increasingly difficult because the right arm pain increases in severity when he lifts his right arm overhead.

6. To further evaluate this patient, you decide to perform a common upper extremity musculoskeletal test. While palpating the radial pulse on his right wrist, you direct the patient to rotate his head to the left and extend it. You have him inhale and hold his breath, and then repeat the procedure with his head rotated and extended to the right side. As you performed this test, you noticed that his radial pulse decreased dramatically on the right side. What is the name of this musculoskeletal test?
   A. Spurling test
   B. Empty can test
   C. Apley scratch test
   D. Hawkins-Kennedy impingement test
   E. Adson test

7. Taking into account the information in question 1, what diagnosis must you include in the differential?
   A. Thoracic outlet syndrome
   B. Rotator cuff tear on the right side
   C. Fractured right radius
   D. Biceps brachii tendonitis on the right side
   E. Anterior glenohumeral laxity on the right side

8. As you are working out at the gym one day, you take notice of your friend who is running on the treadmill. She is breathing heavily, and you remember that as she exhales, she is utilizing which muscles?

   A. Diaphragm.
   B. Scalenes, SCMs, and external intercostals.
   C. Diaphragm, scalenes, SCMs, and external intercostals.
   D. Rectus abdominis, internal and external obliques, transversus abdominis, and internal intercostals.
   E. She is not utilizing any muscles during exhalation because it is always a completely passive process.

9. The next day your friend approaches you and tells you that she has a "stiff neck." She wants to know if there is anything you can do to help her. After a negative workup, you decide to utilize OMT to treat her. You find a couple of anterior cervical CS tenderpoints, and notice that as you palpate in a cephalad to caudad direction, they cross which muscle?

   A. Anterior scalene
   B. Posterior scalene
   C. Middle scalene
   D. Sternocleidomastoid
   E. Trapezius

10. You are now going to treat your friend's anterior cervical tenderpoints, and you remember that, in general, you should position her head in

   A. Flexion, with rotation and sidebending away from the tenderpoint
   B. Extension, with rotation and sidebending away from the tenderpoint
   C. Flexion, with rotation and sidebending toward the tenderpoint
   D. Extension, with rotation and sidebending toward the tenderpoint
   E. Flexion, with rotation toward and sidebending away from the tenderpoint

▶ **ANSWERS**

1. **D**

The thoracic lymphatic pump technique may rupture blebs present in a patient with emphysema. Therefore, if lymph flow needs to be addressed, it is best done using a pedal lymphatic pump technique. The remainder of the choices would be appropriate for this patient.

2. **E**

One would expect to find all of the above SDs in a patient with emphysema who has been coughing recently.

3. **A**

Treatment of C2 may help influence the vagus nerve, which supplies parasympathetic innervation to the diaphragm. Treatment of the thoracic and lumbar spine would be appropriate for normalizing sympathetic tone. The sacrum may affect parasympathetic tone, however, not to the diaphragm.

4. C

There will commonly be a straightforward anatomy question integrated into an OMT question set. Typically, these are not difficult, but you should be prepared for them as these are questions you definitely do not want to miss. The diaphragm is innervated by cervical roots C3, C4, and C5.

5. B

Muscle energy for scalenes is a simple and effective treatment that this patient could do himself while at home. The rest of the answer choices may be difficult or impossible for patients to learn to do on themselves.

6. E

This question is describing Adson test, which is useful in diagnosing thoracic outlet syndrome. Please see Chapter 6 for a complete review of all musculoskeletal tests.

7. A

Taking into account the patient's social history (employment as a window cleaner in which he has his arms extended overhead for long periods of time) as well as the positive Adson test clues us in to the diagnosis. Thoracic outlet syndrome can manifest with symptoms ranging from diffuse arm pain to arm fatigue. It is frequently aggravated by carrying anything in the ipsilateral hand, or by doing overhead work such as painting, window cleaning, or changing a light bulb.

8. D

Since your friend is actively running on a treadmill and breathing heavily, it is safe to say that she is utilizing her secondary muscles of respiration. For exhalation, these muscles include the rectus abdominis, internal and external obliques, transversus abdominis, and internal intercostals. For inhalation, these include scalenes, SCMs, and external intercostals. For primary respiration, only the diaphragm is utilized in inhalation, while exhalation remains completely passive.

9. D

Look at Figure 6-8. The anterior points are located on the anterior surface of the transverse processes of cervical vertebrae; not on the SCM, but the SCM crosses the line of these points.

10. A

In general, anterior cervical CS tenderpoints are treated in flexion, with rotation and sidebending away from the tenderpoint. Whereas posterior cervical CS tenderpoints are treated in extension, with rotation and sidebending away from the tenderpoint. For CS in general, you can remember the pneumonic, "fold and hold." This means you want to *fold* the muscle around the tenderpoint (ie, make it shorter) and *hold* it for approximately 90 seconds.

▶ GASTROENTEROLOGY

Introduction

Osteopathic manipulative technique questions regarding the GI tract typically focus on its relationship to the ANS. Remember that the parasympathetic and sympathetic nervous systems are balanced in the gut. Instead of *increasing* or *decreasing* a specific autonomic influence in the GI tract, therapy should focus on *normalizing* the ANS.

Balance within the ANS is easily achieved. Do not consider whether a technique will increase or decrease a particular autonomic response. Rather, consider whether that technique focuses on the appropriate body region. Note that both diarrhea and constipation affect the vagus nerve, but treating C2 is effective for these two conditions.

Relevant Anatomy

- Foregut—structures from the mouth to the duodenum.
    - Nerve supply—greater splanchnics (T5 to T9)
    - Arterial supply—celiac artery
- Midgut—structures from the duodenum to the proximal two-thirds of the transverse colon.
    - Nerve supply—lesser splanchnics (T10 to T11)
    - Arterial supply—superior mesenteric artery
- Hindgut—structures from the distal one-third of the colon to the anus.
    - Nerve supply—least and lumbar splanchnics (T12 to L2)
    - Arterial supply—inferior mesenteric artery
- Lymphatics—lymphatic drainage of the GI tract is from abdominal trunks that converge to form the cisterna chyli, which then drains to the venous system via the thoracic duct.

Generalized VSR for the GI System

- Sympathetics—T5 to L2
- Parasympathetics—occiput, C1, mainly C2 up to the left colic flexure; S2 to S4 from the left colic flexure to the anus

(For a more specific listing, please refer to Viscerosomatic Reflexes, Chapter 6.)

Osteopathic Considerations and Treatment Guidelines for GI Pathology

Questions on board examinations involving GI disease treatment generally focus on two types of questions.

- What general area of the spine should be treated?
- What GI specific techniques would be appropriate for a given problem?

Example: Diarrhea

- Increased parasympathetic tone
- Increased sympathetic tone secondary to pain
- Treatment guidelines
    - Treat the VSR (normalize autonomic tone).
    - Treat C2 (vagus), pelvic splanchnics (S2-S4)—indirect balancing of C2, sacral rocking
    - Treat the thoracolumbar (TL) junction (T10-L2)—HVLA, ME, CS, ST, DA
    - Chapman reflex points (see Chapter 6)

Similar treatment guidelines can be used to answer the majority of board questions involving the GI tract. Anatomical areas of focus for treating the GI tract should include occiput, atlas, C2, thoracic spine—higher levels for proximal GI tract, lower levels for distal GI tract, lumbar spine at the level of L1 to L2, and the sacrum.

Questions 1–2

A 23-year-old male presents to your clinic after an episode of "food poisoning" 2 weeks ago. He states he recovered without any problem, but has had severe, constant nausea since the episode. After a negative workup, you decide to use OMT as an adjunct treatment.

1. Which of the following treatments would you use for this patient?
    A. Indirect balancing to the upper cervical spine
    B. High velocity, low amplitude for T2
    C. Sternal articulation
    D. Indirect balancing of the sacrum
    E. Muscle energy to the fibular head

2. Where would you expect to find tissue texture changes in this patient?
    A. C2 on the left
    B. C7 on the right
    C. T2 on the right
    D. T3 on the left
    E. Right sacroiliac (SI) joint

Questions 3–5

A 68-year-old female presents to your office 1-year status-post partial colectomy (a portion of the sigmoid colon was removed, specifically) for recurrent diverticulitis. She complains of slight, but uncomfortable, abdominal pain that occurs with certain movements. She saw her surgeon who did a thorough workup but found nothing abnormal.

3. Where would you expect to find tissue texture changes on this patient?
    A. T4 on the right
    B. T7 on the left
    C. T12 on the right
    D. L2 on the left
    E. Over the right ischial tuberosity

4. You decide to try OMT as an adjunct treatment. Which of the following techniques would be appropriate for this patient?
    A. Cervical HVLA
    B. Muscle energy for T2
    C. General lower abdominal/pelvic lift
    D. ME for a forward torsion
    E. Ischiotuberosity spread

5. She also complains of constipation. You decide to treat the parasympathetic autonomics to her affected area. To which region would you direct your treatment?
    A. Occipitomastoid suture
    B. Upper cervical spine
    C. Upper thoracic spine from T1 to T4
    D. Upper lumbar spine
    E. Sacrum

Questions 6–7

6. A 35-year-old female presents to your clinic with recurrent bouts of diarrhea and constipation, as well as abdominal pain for the past 2 years. In addition to doing a thorough history and physical examination, you decide to treat her with OMT. Where would you expect to find CRPs for this patient?
   A. At the tip of the right twelfth rib
   B. Along the iliotibial band (ITB)
   C. Along the intercostal spaces near the sternum
   D. Along the upper thoracic paraspinal areas near the transverse processes
   E. Along the clavicle, first, and second ribs bilaterally

7. At the present time, this patient is suffering from a bout of constipation. Along with treatment of the CRP that you find, you decide to perform an additional osteopathic treatment modality to address her diarrhea. Which modality/modalities would be the most beneficial to treat the parasympathetic autonomics?
   A. Sacral rocking and colonic milking
   B. Paraspinal inhibition of the thoracolumbar junction
   C. High velocity, low amplitude and CS to the upper thoracic spine
   D. Muscle energy to the lumbar spine
   E. Ischial tuberosity spread and colonic milking

Questions 8–10

8. A 47-year-old obese female patient presents to your clinic with abdominal pain that is more prominent on the right than the left. After additional questioning, you learn that the pain is worse with the ingestion of fatty foods. Where would you expect to find tissue texture changes?
   A. T3 to T6 right
   B. T5 to T10 left
   C. T9 to T12 right
   D. T6 to T9 right
   E. T5 to T9 bilaterally

9. The patient from the question above is also complaining of nausea as you interview her. In addition to ordering imaging studies and blood work, you also decide to help treat her symptomatically. To do so, you should utilize which of the following treatments?
   A. Diaphragm release
   B. Colonic milking
   C. Paraspinal inhibition of the thoracolumbar junction
   D. Indirect balancing of the upper cervical spine
   E. Sacral rocking

10. What is the contraindication for performing the treatment selected in question 9?
    A. Arthritis in the cervical spine
    B. An acute asthma attack
    C. An acute UTI
    D. Scoliosis of the thoracic spine
    E. Spondylolisthesis in the lumber spine

1. **A**

Once you hear nausea, you want to think about the vagus nerve. Treating the upper cervical segments, specifically the occiput, atlas, and C2, will be of benefit to this patient. While she could theoretically benefit from any of the above treatments, especially choices A and D, only choice A has an association with the vagus nerve.

2. **A**

Vagus irritability may produce tissue texture changes at the level of C2. While the upper thoracics are thought to produce tissue texture changes in response to cardiac and pulmonary issues, they are not thought to react from issues to the vagus nerve. Nothing in the question stem leaves us to believe this patient is having SI joint problems.

3. **D**

We know this patient had her colon surgically manipulated. Since the highest percentage of diverticula is found in the distal colon, we would expect to find tissue texture changes at the level of L2.

4. **C**

Since this patient has had prior surgery, she may have adhesions or other fascial restrictions in her abdomen. Treating these with an abdominal technique may help free some of these fascial restrictions. Cervical HVLA is probably not a good answer in this case because of the age of the patient. Even if it is completely safe, it is still not addressing her main issue, which is her colon. The same could be said for choices B and D. Choice E may be beneficial but is typically used for lower pelvic organs such as the bladder or prostate. Therefore, the best answer is C.

5. **E**

Again, knowing the anatomic location of this patient's issue and the nervous system that supplies this area gives us our answer. Both the occipitomastoid suture and the upper cervical spine are associated with the vagus nerve; however, the vagus nerve does not innervate the descending and sigmoid colon, where this patient likely had her surgery. The upper thoracic and lumbar spine would be beneficial for modulating sympathetic tone, not parasympathetic tone.

6. **B**

From the history that the patient has given, you should suspect that she has irritable bowel syndrome. The CRPs that correlate with IBS are found on the lower extremity along the ITB. They correlate to the mirror image of the abdominal contents. Answer choice A would be appropriate for appendicitis; C and D for pulmonary pathology; and E for HEENT pathology.

7. **A**

Sacral rocking and colonic milking are both beneficial techniques for this patient because they address the parasympathetic nervous system. Treating the upper thoracic and lumbar spine would be beneficial for modulating sympathetic tone, not parasympathetic tone. While the ischial tuberosity spread may be beneficial, it is typically used for lower pelvic organs such as the bladder and prostate. Therefore, the best answer choice is A.

8. **D**

From this clinical scenario, you should suspect that this patient has some sort of pathology associated with the gallbladder, most likely cholecystitis. You would expect to see tissue texture changes caused by VSR along T6 to T9 on the right, because that is the area associated with the liver and gallbladder. Answer choice A is for the esophagus, B for the stomach, C for the appendix, and E for the pancreas.

9. **D**

This patient will benefit from treatment of the upper cervical spine, most notably the occiput, atlas, and C2 because of their relationship to the vagus nerve. When a patient complains of nausea, always think of the vagus nerve, and when you think of the vagus nerve, think of treating the upper cervicals. Choice A could be beneficial to the patient, although it doesn't necessarily address the nausea issue. Choice B would be beneficial to the patient if she had constipation. Choices C and E could also be beneficial, although sacral rocking and paraspinal inhibition of the thoracolumbar junction would be most appropriate in a patient with diarrhea, not necessarily nausea.

10. **B**

When treating the vagus nerve, vagal stimulation can occur and result in exacerbation of bronchospasm. Do not treat the upper cervicals, most notably C2, during an acute asthma attack. None of the other choices are contraindications to utilizing indirect balancing in the cervical spine. Although choice A can be a contraindication of using HVLA in the cervical spine, arthritis is not a contraindication for indirect balancing of the cervical spine.

▶ UROLOGY AND GYNECOLOGY

Introduction to the Urinary System

Urological dysfunctions can affect all patient populations including men, women, and children. Acute processes must always be assessed before OMT can be used; however, VSR can be used for diagnostic purposes and OMT can be used to treat chronic diseases. As always, board questions tend to focus on VSR and appropriate treatment techniques.

Relevant Anatomy

- Sympathetic innervation of the urinary system
- Kidneys, ureters, bladder: T10 to L1
- Prostate: L1 to L2
- Parasympathetic innervation of the urinary system
- Kidneys, ureters: Very little input to the kidney; the distal ureters get input from S2 to S4
- Bladder and prostate: S2 to S4

Sympathetic VSR for urinary system is at the TL junction.

Generalized VSR of the Urinary System

- Sympathetics—T9 to L2 (think TL junction)
- Parasympathetics—occiput, C1, C2 up to the proximal ureter; S2 to S4 the rest of the way

Osteopathic Considerations and Treatment Guidelines for Urologic Pathology

Examples: Pyelonephritis, renal lithiasis, UTI, benign prostatic hyperplasia (BPH)

- Treat the acute infection with the appropriate medical attention.
- Give pain medication if necessary.
- Use VSR to help with diagnosis.
- Treatment guidelines (when possible):
    - Treat the VSR—ST, Still technique, sacral balancing
    - Treat the pelvic fascia—indirect MFR

Introduction to Gynecology

Pelvic pain affects many women over the course of a lifetime. Pelvic pain may be related to simple dysmenorrhea or to a more complex disease process such as a gynecological neoplasm. Successful pain management comes with a thorough understanding of the relevant anatomy and physiology of the pelvis as well as the innervations of the structures within.

In diagnosing pelvic pain, it is important to identify the dysfunctional area of the pelvic floor. The pelvic floor has three main functions: to support the pelvic organs, to act as a sphincter for perineal openings, and to maintain sexual functions. Pelvic complaints relating to any one of those three functions can guide an osteopathic physician in terms of treatment.

Gynecological questions on the boards involving OMM focus on VSR and treatment for common gynecological pathology. A brief overview of pelvic and other gynecological complaints will be discussed as well as their associated SD and appropriate treatment guidelines.

Relevant Anatomy

- Pelvic floor
    - Muscles: Levator ani muscles and pelvic diaphragm complex
    - Contains: Visceral pelvic fascia, pelvic diaphragm, deep genital muscles, sphincter muscles
- Autonomic innervation of pelvic organs (ovaries, fallopian tubes, uterus, cervix, vagina)
    - Sympathetic—T9 to L1
    - Parasympathetic—S2 to S4

Generalized VSR for the Pelvic Organs

- Sympathetics—T9 to L1
- Parasympathetics—S2 to S4

    (For a more specific list, please refer to Chapter 6.)

Osteopathic Considerations and Treatment Guidelines for Gynecological Pathology

DYSMENORRHEA

- Causes: Uterine contractions, ischemia, chronic pain syndromes, or other psychological disorders affecting pain perception, cervical pathology (cervical stenosis).
    - Determine whether it is primary or secondary.

*Think outside the pelvis–treat
the thoracics too!*

- Manifestations: Painful menstruation, cramping, nausea, fatigue, headache
- VSR: T10 to L1, S2 to S4
- Treatment guidelines
  - Chapman points within the ITB may be present; treatment of these points may be beneficial.
  - Lymphatic techniques: Edema and bloating can be associated with dysmenorrhea; focus on treating the upper thoracics and the thoracic outlet (may alleviate breast tenderness as well).
  - Sacral techniques: Inhibitory pressure can decrease uterine contractions and is well-tolerated.

PREMENSTRUAL SYNDROME

- Causes: (not limited to) Hormonal imbalances, psychological, social, or genetic factors, vitamin deficiencies
- Manifestations: Bloating, weight gain, irritability, mood changes, fatigue
- VSR: T9 to L1, S2 to S4, C2 (vagus) may be present
- Treatment guidelines
  - Treat the VSR.
  - Treat lymphatics.
  - Check for OA dysfunction.
  - Lumbosacral decompression.
  - Sacral techniques: Rocking of the sacral base helps to inhibit the parasympathetics.

*Sacral rocking inhibits
parasympathetics to the pelvic
organs.*

PELVIC FLOOR DYSFUNCTION

- Causes: (not limited to) Pregnancy, labor trauma, weakness of muscular structures, previous sexual abuse, pelvic structural trauma
- Manifestations: Incontinence (fecal and urinary), sexual dysfunction, prolapse of pelvic organs, dyspareunia
- VSR: T9 to L1, S2 to S4
- Treatment guidelines
  - Trigger points (not tenderpoints) are found in many of the muscular structures including coccygeus, levator ani, obturator internus, adductor magnus, and piriformis.
  - Counterstrain and MFR techniques can be very beneficial.
  - Direct inhibitory pressure of intravaginal structures.
  - Pelvic diaphragm release.

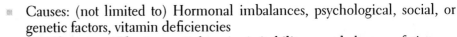

▶ REVIEW QUESTIONS: UROLOGY

1. A 26-year-old female complains of burning with urination and urgency. You start her on Cipro 250 mg twice a day for 3 days. You also assess and treat the VSR at the level of
   - A. C2
   - B. T1 to T3
   - C. T6 to T8
   - D. T12 to L1
   - E. L4 to L5

2. A 77-year-old female presents with severe low back pain, fever/chills, and dysuria for the past week. You order a urine culture that shows *Escherichia coli* and a urine sample that shows leukocyte casts with hematuria. You also note tissue texture change at which level?
   A. C2
   B. T1 to T3
   C. T6 to T8
   D. T12 to L1
   E. L4 to L5

3. A 62-year-old healthy male complains of difficulty maintaining a steady stream of urine for the past few months. He denies dysuria and fevers. The urinalysis is negative. You find tissue texture change at the level of T12 to L2. What should be at the top of your differential diagnosis?
   A. Pyelonephritis
   B. Benign prostatic hyperplasia
   C. Urinary tract infection (UTI)
   D. Renal lithiasis
   E. Cystitis

► ANSWERS

1, **D.** 2, **D.** 3, **B.**

All of these questions refer to the VSR for the urinary system. Question 1 addresses the bladder affected by a UTI. Question 2 addresses the kidneys affected by pyelonephritis. Question 3 addresses the prostate affected by BPH.

► REVIEW QUESTIONS: GYNECOLOGY

Questions 1–2

A 32-year-old female, G2P2002, presents to her gynecologist and states that her husband requested that she do something about her premenstrual syndrome (PMS). She states that her symptoms of irritability and mood changes are "getting worse" throughout the past few years and she would like some relief.

1. Which areas do you expect to find VSR?
   A. C2 and T1 to T4
   B. C2 and T5 to T9
   C. C2 and L3 to L5
   D. S2 to S4 and T9 to L1
   E. S2 to S4 and L3 to L5

2. The gynecologist starts the patient on oral contraceptive pills (OCPs) and decides to do OMT. Which of the following techniques is most appropriate for relieving symptoms of PMS?
   A. Sacral rocking
   B. Indirect balancing of the diaphragm
   C. Rib raising
   D. Muscle energy for a rotated ilium
   E. Frontal lift

Questions 3–4

A 19-year-old female, gravida 0, para 0 (G0P0), complains of painful cramping associated with every menstrual cycle. She began her menses at age 12; her cycles are every 32 days and they last for 7 days. A Pap smear was done and her pelvic examination is normal.

3. What area of the body do you expect to find CRPs?
   A. Posterior cervical spine
   B. Costosternal joints
   C. Medial border of the scapula
   D. Thoracolumbar junction
   E. Iliotibial band

4. You decide to treat the patient with inhibitory pressure of the sacrum. This technique most improves dysmenorrhea by
   A. Affecting the sympathetics to the pelvic organs
   B. Decreasing uterine contractions
   C. Increasing levels of circulating estrogen
   D. Affecting the Jones' CS tenderpoint of the iliolumbar ligament
   E. Leveling the sacral base

5. A 56-year-old female, with four previous normal spontaneous vaginal deliveries (NSVDs) presents to your office with complaints of incontinence. Her symptoms started about a year ago, but she now admits that she has recently started using absorbent pads. You diagnose her with a prolapsed bladder. The patient wants to avoid surgery. Aside from medical treatment, what OMT can be used to help with her symptoms?
   A. Muscle energy of the TL junction
   B. Indirect balancing of C2
   C. Cervical ST
   D. Counterstrain of anterior L5 tenderpoint
   E. Muscle energy of psoas

▶ **ANSWERS**

1. **D**

Sometimes OMM questions on the boards do not directly address musculoskeletal issues. When presented with a gynecology case, regardless of the signs and symptoms, think VSR. For the pelvic organs, the sympathetics are at the TL junction (T9-L1). The parasympathetics are at S2 to S4. Specifically for PMS, the vagus reflex at C2 may be present secondary to manifestations of abdominal complaints such as cramping and diarrhea.

2. **A**

Sacral rocking is a technique that affects the pelvic splanchnics (S2-S4). These are the VSR for parasympathetic innervation of the pelvic organs. Balancing the diaphragm helps with respiratory complaints. Rib raising helps to decrease sympathetic tone. The patient may have some unrelated ilium dysfunction, which may respond to ME, but this technique would not specifically help with the symptoms of PMS. Frontal lift primarily affects the sinuses.

3. E

Patients with dysmenorrhea have pelvic visceral irritation, which can manifest in CRP in the ITB. All the other regions listed are not associated with pelvic complaints. Posterior cervical spine, HEENT; the costosternal joints, respiratory pathology; medial border of the scapula, upper extremity complaints; TL junction, adrenal pathology.

4. B

Inhibitory pressure of the sacrum directly affects the parasympathetics to the pelvic organs, specifically the uterus. This results in a decrease of uterine contractions, which can improve dysmenorrhea. None of the sympathetic innervation of any organ comes from the sacrum. This technique plays no role in the hormonal regulation of estrogen nor does it treat the iliolumbar ligament, which doesn't contribute to dysmenorrhea regardless. Leveling the sacral base alone will not improve dysmenorrhea.

5. A

This patient has pelvic floor dysfunction most likely because of her four vaginal deliveries. Treating the TL junction will directly affect the sympathetics not only to the pelvic organs but also to the organs of the urinary system (kidneys, bladder). Normalizing autonomic tone to this region will not fix her prolapsed bladder, but may allow for better control of her urine. Treating C2 or the other cervical vertebrae have no effect on this area. This patient may have an anterior L5 tenderpoint or a tight psoas, but treating neither will help to balance the ANS.

▶ OBSTETRICS

Introduction

A pregnant woman's SD can change dramatically over the 40 weeks of pregnancy. Therefore, regular screening structural examinations are essential throughout pregnancy, not only to identify new SD, but also to address worsening chronic SD. Life-threatening maternal and fetal medical concerns must be addressed early at each patient encounter, but a structural examination and OMT should be an integral part of every visit.

Obstetrics questions on the boards involving OMM tend to focus on VSR and treatment guidelines throughout the different trimesters. Remember, as a woman's body develops over the course of a pregnancy, so will her diagnosis and treatment.

Relevant Anatomy and Overview of Changes during Pregnancy

MUSCULOSKELETAL

- Increased lordosis and change in the center of gravity (Figure 5-1).
- Compensatory increase in the thoracic kyphosis.
- Abdominal muscles become overstretched while the paraspinal muscles become shortened and tight.
- Possible exacerbation of scoliosis.
- Changes in contour of the rib cage affecting respiration.
- Radicular symptoms of extremities secondary to the uterus placing pressure on the nerve roots of the lumbosacral spine.

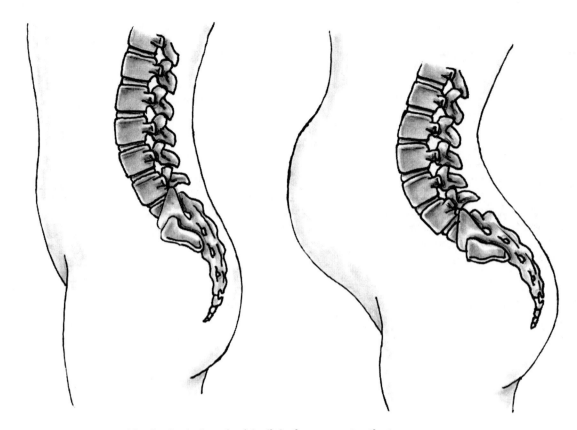

FIGURE 5-1. Increased lumbar lordosis and pelvic tilt in the pregnant patient.

Lymphatics may be at the root of many manifestations of pregnancy.

There are additional VSRs that come late with specific manifestations of pregnancy.

LYMPHATICS AND OTHER FLUIDS

- Circulation to the pelvis increases in order to support the existing pregnancy.
- An imbalance exists between the increased fluid in the pelvis and the decrease in return of the fluid to the systemic circulation leading to pelvic floor congestion.
- Decreased fluid return also results in upper and lower extremity congestion and edema, which in turn may cause problems in the extremities.

HORMONAL

- Relaxin is released which allows the maternal pelvic ligaments to accommodate the growing fetus.
- Ligamentous laxity is present throughout the whole body, but can lead to hypermobility, especially in the SI joints, pubic symphysis, and hips.
- Increased levels of progesterone can cause HAs, nausea, decreased peristalsis of the GI tract, and can affect the thoracic cage leading to an increase in tidal volume.

Generalized VSR for the Pelvic Organs

- Sympathetics—T9 to L2
- Parasympathetics—S2 to S4

(For a complete listing, see Chapter 6.)

Osteopathic Considerations and Treatment Guidelines for the Pregnant Patient

FIRST TRIMESTER

The sacrum should be a primary treatment focus during the first trimester. Improved sacral symmetry and motion during the early stages of pregnancy will make new-onset SD easier to treat. Both indirect and direct techniques can be used. Any treatment position comfortable for the patient is appropriate, including the prone position.

MANIFESTATIONS OF FIRST-TRIMESTER PREGNANCY AND RELATED SD

Hyperemesis

- Cause: Not exactly understood.
- VSR: C2 on the left (vagus reflex), T5 to T9 (additional GI discomfort).
- Treatment guidelines: Decrease suboccipital tension with MFR (killer fingers); treat C2 with indirect balancing; treat C3 to C5 (phrenic nerve); treat the upper thoracics with ST, HVLA, ME, CS.

Pelvic Floor Congestion

- Cause: Increased circulation to the pelvic organs and decreased venous return to the systemic circulation.
- Treatment guidelines: Ischial tuberosity spread, lymphatic pedal pump, range of motion (ROM) exercises of the lower extremities.

Sacral Dysfunction

- As mentioned above, any sacral dysfunction should be treated in the first trimester. All sacral techniques can be used.

SECOND TRIMESTER

During the second trimester, hyperemesis often resolves, but the patient is at risk for developing other complications. The clinician should continue to treat all SDs, related and unrelated to the pregnancy. Both indirect and direct techniques are most useful. The patient can be treated in any position including the prone position.

MANIFESTATIONS OF SECOND-TRIMESTER PREGNANCY AND RELATED SD

Round Ligament Pain

- Cause: As the gravid uterus becomes larger, there is increased tension of the round ligaments, which can cause pain, cramping, and discomfort in the lower abdominal area.
- VSR: T10 to L1.
- Treatment guidelines: Direct or indirect MFR of the abdominal fascia, anterior lumbar CS tenderpoints L3 to L5 (correlates with round ligament pain).

Carpal Tunnel

- Cause: Increased localized edema and swelling in the carpal tunnel; can be attributed to breast congestion, axillary congestion, and changes in the postural mechanics of the head and neck.

A tenderpoint in pronator teres muscle is often present in carpal tunnel.

- Treatment guidelines: Myofascial release of the thoracic outlet; treat the axial component in the upper thoracics; CS in the forearm (median nerve travels through pronator teres where a tenderpoint may be present); MFR of the carpel tunnel.
- Night splints may be necessary.
- Often resolves after delivery.

THIRD TRIMESTER

The female body endures the most stress during the third trimester. The lumbar lordosis increases, venous flow decreases, and the patient can become structurally fatigued. Again, depending on the situation, both indirect and direct techniques can still be used. Most techniques should be performed with the patient seated or lying on her side. Remember to place the female on her left side during the sidelying techniques so the fetus does not compress the inferior vena cava (IVC) further. Continue treating the general VSR.

MANIFESTATIONS OF THIRD-TRIMESTER PREGNANCY AND RELATED SD

Lower Extremity Edema and Hemorrhoids

- Cause: As the pelvic contents continue to enlarge and gravity takes an effect, more and more pressure is placed on the venous and lymphatic return from the lower extremities as well as the IVC, which leads to increased venous congestion.
- Treatment guidelines: Any type of myofascial technique used to increase lymphatic flow; treat the SD that corresponds with the viscerosomatic (VS) reflexes; treat the pelvic diaphragm to lift pelvic contents.

Reflux

> **Remember the common GI pattern for reflux.**
>
> - C2L
> - T3R
> - T5L
> - T7R

- Cause: Can be structural (ie, compression of the abdominal contents) or hormonal (ie, relaxation of the lower esophageal sphincter).
- VSR: Gastrointestinal pattern (C2 left, T3 right, T5 left, T7 right); in general, focus on T5 to T9 and C2 (vagus).
- Treatment guidelines: High velocity, low amplitude to midthoracics (ie, epigastric thrust), indirect balancing of C2; treatment of the respiratory diaphragm.

CONSIDERATIONS OF OMT DURING LABOR

OMT can still be used throughout labor. This will largely depend on the condition of the patient.

- Gentle techniques are tolerated well, especially in early labor.
- Treating the sympathetics can induce labor, while treating the parasympathetics can induce cervical dilation.
- Cranial techniques have been shown to influence contractions.
- Absolutely no direct or otherwise aggressive treatments; fetal well-being must always be kept in mind.

SD DIRECTLY RELATED TO TRAUMA OF DELIVERY

Most of the structural trauma is related to the way in which the fetus travels through the birth canal. Significant strain is placed upon the pelvis and ST, which can persist after delivery.

- Iliac dysfunction—up-slip or down-slip of the ilium; anterior or posterior ilium; pubic symphysis dysfunction/separation
- Sacral base restriction—either torsions or shears
- Lumbosacral junction dysfunction—disc pathology
- Lower extremity neuropathy associated with lower back trauma

CONTRAINDICATIONS OF OMT IN THE PREGNANT PATIENT

Table 5-1 outlines contraindications by trimester.

POSTPARTUM CONSIDERATIONS

The goal of treatment during the postpartum period is to return the patient to her pregravid state. Breast-feeding mothers may have continued upper thoracic pain and carpal tunnel symptoms. Techniques used to address these problems during pregnancy can absolutely be used during the postpartum time.

TABLE 5-1. Contraindications of OMT in the Pregnant Patient Divided by Trimester

PATHOLOGY	FIRST TRIMESTER	SECOND TRIMESTER	THIRD TRIMESTER
Vaginal bleeding of unknown etiology	X	X	X
History of recent abdominal trauma	X	X	X
Ectopic pregnancy	X		
Possibility of threatened or incomplete abortion	X	X	
Placenta previa		X	X
Abruption		X	X
PROM		X	X
PTL		X	X
Prolapsed umbilical cord			X
Pre-eclampsia/eclampsia/ pregnancy-induced hypertension		X	X

OMT, osteopathic manipulative techniques; PROM, premature rupture of membranes; PTL, preterm labor.

137

Questions 1–3

A 27-year-old female, G1P0 at 9 and 3/7 weeks, presents for an initial prenatal visit. An ultrasound (US) confirms an intrauterine pregnancy (IUP) and the patient has an enlarged uterus upon palpation.

1. The patient is complaining of morning sickness. Where are you most likely to palpate VSR?
   A. C2
   B. T1 to T3
   C. T11 to T12
   D. L3 to L5
   E. S2 to S4

2. Which technique is most appropriate to treat her symptoms of nausea?
   A. Sacral inhibitory pressure
   B. Counterstrain of iliolumbar ligament
   C. Direct treatment of inhaled ribs
   D. Soft tissue of the upper thoracics
   E. Muscle energy of the mid to lower thoracics

3. The structural examination reveals a low anterior superior iliac spine (ASIS) on the right, a low posterior superior iliac spine (PSIS) on the left, and restriction of motion of the right ilium. Standing flexion test is positive on the right. What type of SD does she most likely have?
   A. Posterior ilium on the right
   B. Left innominate up-slip
   C. Posterior sacrum on the left
   D. Anterior ilium on the right
   E. Unilaterally extended sacrum on the left

Questions 4–5

A 31-year-old female, G2P1 at 22 and 1/7 weeks, presents to the OB clinic with complaints of numbness and tingling in her right hand. She has never had this before, and her symptoms only started a few weeks ago. Upon examination, her uterus is measuring at 21 cm and fetal heart tones (FHT) are in the 130s. The upper extremity examination reveals a positive Phalen test and a positive Tinel sign of the right hand. You diagnose carpal tunnel.

4. What is the most likely cause of carpal tunnel in the second trimester of pregnancy?
   A. Compression of the IVC by the fetus
   B. Breast and axillary congestion
   C. Increased lumbar lordosis
   D. Flexed dysfunctions in the TL junction
   E. Restriction of the hemidiaphragm

5. Aside from utilizing night splints to relieve the symptoms, what osteopathic technique would be most appropriate to treat the patient?
   A. HVLA of the upper cervicals
   B. CS of levator scapulae
   C. MFR of the thoracic outlet

D. CS of the biceps tendon

E. ME of the TL junction

6. During the first trimester, the most important treatment to focus on is:

A. Relieving pressure from an increased lumbar lordosis

B. Myofascial release of the carpal tunnel

C. Normalization of the sacrum

D. Abdominal release for a hiatal hernia

E. Generalized myofascial techniques to improve lymphatic flow

▶ ANSWERS

1. A

Hyperemesis in the first trimester is a very common problem of pregnancy. The nausea associated with it will cause a VSR of the vagus nerve (parasympathetic innervation to the gut) resulting in SD of C2. Other VSR: T1 to T3—cardiac or pulmonary, T11 to T12—genitourinary (GU), L3 to L5—no VSR, S2 to S4—parasympathetics of lower GI and GU.

2. E

The sympathetic innervation of the gut comes from T5 to T9. Muscle energy is an appropriate technique to treat this area. All of the other areas of treatment do not have an effect on nausea or other GI symptoms.

3. D

A standing structural examination is very important to do as early on in the pregnancy as possible. The positive standing flexion test on the right immediately clues you in to a problem with the ilium on the right. The low ASIS on the right and restriction of motion on the right confirms your diagnosis of an anterior ilium on the right.

4. B

During the second trimester, increased breast and axillary congestion lead to localized edema and swelling throughout the upper extremity. Compression of the IVC typically does not occur until later pregnancy (third trimester). Structural changes of the TL junction and lumbar spine may be present, but do not contribute directly to carpal tunnel.

5. C

MFR of the thoracic outlet will facilitate drainage of the venous and lymphatic systems of the upper extremity. While SD may be present in many other areas of the body, treatment of these areas will not directly affect the thoracic outlet.

6. C

Normalizing the sacrum and keeping it functioning properly as the mother's body changes is of key importance in the first trimester.

▶ PEDIATRICS

Introduction

The pediatric patient can frequently present to the physician's office with complaints that go undiagnosed. Many dysfunctions are related to trauma from birth. Other dysfunctions occur from injuries secondary to repetitive postural patterns. The musculoskeletal system of the pediatric patient is more flexible than that of the adult caused by the greater ratio of cartilage to bone. This allows for more frequent dysfunctions because the skeletal system is not rigid. However, it allows techniques like cranial manipulation, indirect balancing, ME, and FPR to work well in resolving SD. The skeletal system has yet to develop fully. Using a strong force can be detrimental.

Relevant Anatomy

CRANIAL

(See Figure 5-2.)

- Made up of the cranial base and vault.
- The vault has areas of ossification within membranous areas.
- The base is made up of fibrocartilaginous articulations.
- The cartilaginous and membranous portions, which permit maximum compressibility, allow the fetus' head to move through the birth canal.

Osteopathic Considerations and Treatment Guidelines or the Pediatric Patient

CRANIAL DYSFUNCTIONS

The following cranial dysfunctions are typically attributed to birth trauma. Most dysfunctions can be treated in similar ways using various craniosacral techniques (please refer to Chapter 7).

ANTERIOR OCCIPUT

- Results in compression of the twelfth cranial nerve (hypoglossal nerve)
- Manifestations: Problems with the suckling mechanism

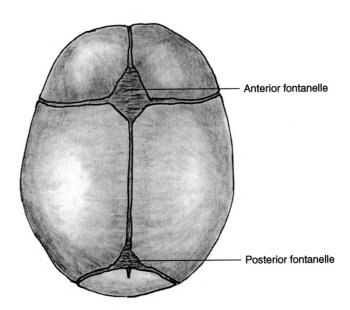

FIGURE 5-2. Pediatric cranium.

- Can also occur after birth if the baby is constantly held in the same position while feeding (slight left lateral decubitus position with the head turned left and flexed)
- Treatment guidelines: Craniosacral techniques

MISSHAPED HEAD

- Cause: Sphenobasilar lateral strain as the baby is moving through the mother's pelvic girdle (birth canal)
- Manifestations
  - Parallelogram-shaped head
  - Entrapment of CN III, IV, and VI, which can cause eye dysfunction
- Treatment guidelines: Craniosacral techniques

CONE-SHAPED HEAD

- Cause: Increased time in the birth canal or vacuum extraction.
- Manifestations: The entire cranial vault becomes disproportionate.
- Treatment guidelines: Craniosacral techniques.

OTHER COMMON PEDIATRIC PATHOLOGY

TORTICOLLIS

(See Figure 5-3.)

- Cause: Unilateral contraction of the SCM
- Manifestations
  - The infant's neck is sidebent and rotated in opposite directions.
  - Temporal dysfunction secondary to attachments of SCM.
  - The SCM originates from the manubrium (sternal head) and medial portion of the clavicle (clavicular head) and inserts on the mastoid process of the temporal bone.
- Treatment guidelines
  - Craniosacral techniques
  - Indirect techniques of the cervical spine and clavicle
  - Counterstrain of SCM

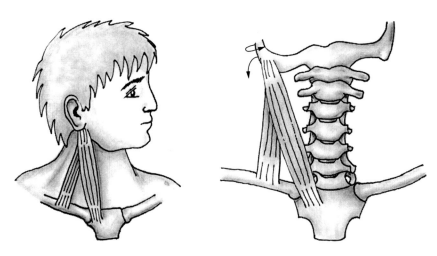

FIGURE 5-3. Torticollis: tight right SCM.

PELVIC GIRDLE DYSFUNCTION

- Cause: Strain during birth or growth plate development
- Manifestations: Craniosacral dysfunction, asymmetric rotation of the innominates, genu varus/valgus, short leg syndrome, scoliosis
- Treatment guidelines
  - Craniosacral techniques
  - Treatment of the ilium—ME, indirect balancing of the pelvis

▶ REVIEW QUESTIONS: PEDIATRICS

Questions 1–5

A concerned mother brings her 8-week-old infant in to the clinic. She would like to know if there is anything else that can be done to improve the overall health of her child. In addition to counseling on diet and safety, you decide to treat the infant using OMT.

1. The mother states that her previous child had trouble with suckling as an infant, even though his appetite was good. You explain to her that a possible cause for this may have been _____ compressing the _____.
   A. Condylar compression, twelfth nerve
   B. Diaphragm restriction, esophagus
   C. Inguinal hernia, genitofemoral nerve
   D. Umbilical hernia, small intestine
   E. Psoas hypertrophy, SI joint

2. The mother then tells you this child had a parallelogram-shaped head when she was born. What cranial strain pattern would you suspect?
   A. Torsion
   B. Sidebending rotation
   C. Lateral strain
   D. Vertical strain
   E. Sphenobasilar synchondrosis compression

3. While treating the infant, the mother tells you about a friend of hers who had a child with torticollis. Which CN would you suspect was involved?
   A. III
   B. IV
   C. VII
   D. IX
   E. XI

4. Which cranial bone may become dysfunctional as a result of torticollis?
   A. Frontal
   B. Sphenoid
   C. Parietal
   D. Temporal
   E. Occiput

5. While palpating the infant in the vault hold, you note that the rate and amplitude of the cranial rhythmic impulse (CRI) seem decreased. What other anatomic region would be helpful in addressing the CRI?
   A. C2
   B. Upper thoracic spine

C. Lumbar spine
D. Sacrum
E. Fibular head

6. Common pediatric dysfunctions that are treatable by craniosacral therapy include all of the following except
   A. Torticollis
   B. Parallelogram-shaped head
   C. Pelvic girdle dysfunction
   D. Cleft palate
   E. Condylar compression

▶ ANSWERS

1. A

Condylar compression is the most likely of the above choices given the anatomy of the occiput at birth. Compression of the twelfth nerve could have produced difficulty with suckling. The remainder of the choices would have produced additional symptoms in addition to suckling difficulties.

2. C

Whenever you see "parallelogram" in a question pertaining to cranial strain patterns, you should immediately think of lateral strains. None of the other choices would produce a parallelogram-shaped head.

3. E

Cranial nerve XI is typically the culprit in torticollis, causing dysfunction of the SCM. The remaining CNs may produce other systemic dysfunctions if irritated, but would not affect the SCM muscle.

4. D

Tension on the mastoid process as a result from a hypertonic SCM may produce temporal bone dysfunction. This could lead to dysfunction of the remainder of the cranial bones; however, the temporal bone would be the primary bone affected in torticollis.

5. D

Pelvic girdle dysfunction is common after birth. Sacral dysfunction may be responsible for the decreased rate and amplitude of the CRI. Therefore, treatment of the sacrum may help improve the cranial mechanism.

6. D

Cleft palate (which often occurs along with clefting of the lip) is a congenital deformity caused by abnormal facial development during gestation. It may be improved by craniosacral technique, but this deformity is not an example of SD and is treatable by surgery.

▶ THE HOSPITALIZED AND POSTSURGICAL PATIENT

Introduction

Patients that have been hospitalized, and more specifically, those who are postsurgical are compromised in some way. It may be decreased lung function because of a recent coronary artery bypass graft (CABG) or decreased ROM secondary to immobilization of a fracture. Regardless of the situation, certain concepts need to be kept in mind when using OMT. Determining a goal of treatment helps to decipher which techniques are appropriate. The different types of treatment tend to be a focus on the boards.

Osteopathic Considerations and Treatment Guidelines for the Hospitalized or Postoperative Patient

GOALS OF TREATMENT AND EXAMPLES OF SPECIFIC TECHNIQUES

(Not all-inclusive)

- Increase venous and lymphatic return/decrease edema and congestion
  - Extremity ROM exercises
  - Lymphatic techniques—pedal pump, lymphatic pump
  - Myofascial release of the thoracic outlet
- Increase ROM (muscles and joints)/decrease edema
  - Range of motion exercises
- Normalize the ANS
  - Treat VSR
  - Rib raising
  - Sacral rocking
- Normalize the CRI
  - Craniosacral techniques
- Increase lung function
  - Treat the VSR—indirect techniques of the upper thoracics, ST, CS
  - Indirect balancing of the diaphragm
  - Rib techniques—CS, balancing
- Stimulate the bowels
  - Rib raising
  - Treat the mid-lower thoracics

EXAMPLE OF POSTOPERATIVE SURGICAL CASE WITH APPROPRIATE TECHNIQUES

CORONARY ARTERY BYPASS GRAFT

- Early stages—*no* HVLA; rib raising, cervical ST (focus on C2—vagus), early mobilization (walking)
- Later stages—sternal articulation, rib walking, treat the upper thoracics (ME, CS, DA)

> ► **REVIEW QUESTIONS: THE HOSPITALIZED PATIENT/POSTSURGICAL PATIENT**

1. A 55-year-old female presents to her primary care physician for the first time in several years. She has smoked 1 pack of cigarettes a day for 35 years. She now complains of an intermittent, productive cough and dyspnea that has bothered her for the last 2 years. The physician suspects chronic obstructive pulmonary disease (COPD). On the musculoskeletal examination of the thoracic cage, he expects to find
   A. T5, sidebent right, rotated right, and flexed
   B. Decreased thoracic motion in exhalation
   C. An elevated first rib on the left side
   D. Increased compliance of the thoracic cage
   E. Decreased thoracic motion in inhalation

2. A 75-year-old male is hospitalized for an acute exacerbation of congestive heart failure (CHF). After a thorough evaluation, you and your attending physician think that OMT might be beneficial to the patient. Your first step before performing OMT is to
   A. Place the patient in a completely supine position
   B. Call the patient's family to request consent
   C. Determine which techniques may be most appropriate
   D. Perform a complete physical examination
   E. Determine the patient's urine output

3. Release of the respiratory diaphragm and employment of the pedal pump technique both serve to
   A. Increase fluid movement throughout the body
   B. Quiet VSR
   C. Mobilize the thoracic cage
   D. Exacerbate cardiac arrhythmias
   E. Increase the likelihood of a local inflammatory reaction

4. While on your surgery rotation, you round on a patient who is 48 hours post-CABG. Your attending physician would like you to perform OMT to help aid in his recovery. What technique would be most appropriate?
   A. Myofascial release to the thoracic inlet
   B. Articulation to the thoracic cage
   C. Thoracic pump
   D. Rib raising
   E. All of the above

5. The above patient is now 2 months post-CABG. Which OMT technique would be most appropriate at this time?
   A. Myofascial release to the thoracic inlet
   B. Articulation to the thoracic cage
   C. Thoracic pump
   D. Rib raising
   E. All of the above

▶ ANSWERS

1. **B**

COPD is considered an obstructive lung disease. As a result, patients will generally present with limited thoracic cage motion during exhalation. Limited motion may be palpated on the musculoskeletal examination.

2. **C**

Osteopathic manipulative techniques for the hospitalized patient must be individualized to the patient's illness and needs. Of paramount importance is determining which techniques will be most appropriate for this patient.

3. **A**

A tense diaphragm can constrict the thoracic duct. Decreased diaphragmatic movement will decrease the intrathoracic/intra-abdominal pressure gradient. The pedal pump technique indirectly massages the thoracic duct through increased frequency of the movement of fascia and viscera.

4. A

In someone who is 48 hours postoperative, only very gentle techniques would be appropriate. While the rest of the techniques would help mobilize lymph and normalize sympathetic tone, they may also inhibit healing by placing undue strain on a fragile thoracic cage, which has been recently opened and is now reconnected with wires.

5. E

Enough time has now passed to give the thoracic cage a chance to heal; therefore, any of the above techniques would be appropriate and helpful to this patient.

SECTION IV

Historical Highlights, Key Points, and Musculoskeletal Tests

▶ High-Yield Topics
for the COMLEX

High-Yield Topics for the COMLEX

Occasionally, the Comprehensive Osteopathic Medical Licensing Examination (COMLEX) asks historical questions. Included in the following section is a list of important historical events. Viscerosomatic reflexes (VSR), Chapman reflex points (CRP), and Jones' counterstrain (CS) tenderpoints are commonly included as adjunct questions to clinical scenarios. The following section also contains this information in a table format. Use these tables as a quick review the night before the examination.

▶ HISTORY OF OSTEOPATHY

- 1828: A.T. Still was born in Virginia.
- 1874: A.T. Still "flung to the breeze the banner of osteopathy."
- 1892: American School of Osteopathy (ASO) opens in Kirksville, Missouri.
- 1893: Nettie Bolles is the first woman to serve on an Osteopathic Faculty—an example of A.T. Still's commitment to women's rights.
- 1896: Vermont is the first state to recognize osteopathy.
- 1897: American Osteopathic Association (AOA) is founded—originally the American Association for the Advancement of Osteopathy.
- 1898: Second college founded—Philadelphia College and Infirmary of Osteopathy (will become PCOM).
- 1899: William Smith, MD, ASO faculty, first to delineate the arterial system with x-rays. First and only x-ray west of Mississippi. Mark Twain testifies on behalf of osteopathy to help obtain practice rights in New York.
- 1900: J. Martin Littlejohn, MD, DO, founded the American College of Osteopathic Medicine and Surgery in Chicago.
- 1905: Des Moines College founded.
- 1916: Kansas City College founded. No new colleges until 1966.
- 1917: The profession mounts an effort to gain federal recognition and the right to serve in the uniformed services.
- 1910: The Flexner report. A scathing report on medical and osteopathic education by Abraham Flexner of the Rockefeller Institute. As a result of this report, many allopathic and osteopathic colleges were closed. This report forced the AOA to develop standards for teaching osteopathy in colleges and lead to AOA accreditation.
- 1918: H.H. Fryette, DO, introduces his concepts of spinal motion. He gives to the profession the development of the articulated spine and the principles of spinal motion (Principle I and II).
- 1936: The Applied Academy of Osteopathy (AAO) is formed from the Osteopathic Manipulative Therapeutic and Clinical Research Association.
- 1939: William G. Sutherland, DO, DSc (hon), proposed the cranial concept.
- 1944: The name AAO is changed to American Academy of Osteopathy. H.H. Fryette, DO, publishes his text *Principles of Osteopathic Technique*.
- 1950: Dr. Angus Cathie forms the first Undergraduate American Academy of Osteopathy (UAAO) at PCOM.
- 1950s: Lawrence Jones, DO, develops his technique known as strain/CS.
- 1955: Fred Mitchell Sr, DO, introduces his muscle energy technique.
- 1962: Licensing of osteopathic physicians in California is halted. MD degrees are granted to DOs for the fee of $65. Nearly 2000 of California's 2400 DOs become MDs. The Los Angeles College of Osteopathic Physicians and Surgeons becomes an allopathic medical school.
- 1963: DOs are accepted by the civil service as medical officers on equal footing with MDs.
- 1966: Robert McNamara, Secretary of Defense, directs the Army, Navy, and Air Force to accept qualified DOs as medical officers.

- **1970:** Most colleges changed names to "college of osteopathic medicine." Allopathic postdoctoral training opens to DOs.
- **1971:** Michigan State University College of Osteopathic Medicine founded first university-affiliated and state-funded college. The California State Supreme Court restores licensure of osteopathic physicians.
- **1994:** Judith O'Connell, DO, represents the osteopathic profession before the AMA's committee on CPT codes. She successfully argues to have specific procedure codes for osteopathic manipulative treatment accepted and included in the national coding manual.
- **2004:** 22 colleges of osteopathic medicine.
- **2008:** 25 colleges of osteopathic medicine in 28 locations.

▶ VISCEROSOMATIC REFLEXES

The COMLEX loves to include VSR questions. They are commonly added at the end of specific case scenarios and serve to challenge osteopathic diagnostic skills. For convenience, a complete list of VSR is found in Table 6-1. The list is comprehensive but for high-yield study purposes should be understood regionally. Following the table are groupings of VSR (primarily sympathetic) for the different organ systems. Remembering approximately what area of the body corresponds with a particular system will help rule out the distracters on test day.

Introduction

Viscerosomatic reflexes are a type of somatic dysfunction (SD) caused by changes in the autonomic nervous system (ANS) (see Figure 6-1). They can be acute or chronic and are considered a somatic representation of visceral disease. When either branch of the ANS continuously overstimulates a particular organ, a reflex reaction occurs. The soma at the same level of the organ's autonomic innervation takes on characteristics of SD (Tissue texture change **A**symmetry **R**estriction of motion **T**enderness [**TART**]). The degree of SD is directly related to the degree of visceral pathology.

Sympathetic nervous system– think thoracolumbar. Parasympathetic nervous system–think craniosacral.

- Sympathetic nervous system.
  - Enhances or accelerates the activity of organs
  - Arises from the thoracolumbar spinal segments
- Parasympathetic nervous system.
  - Inhibits or decelerates the activity of organs.
  - Arises from the craniosacral area of the spine.
  - **High cervicals (C0-C2) are also included, particularly C2 on the left, which is specific for cranial nerve (CN) X, vagus. (Know this vagus reflex. It's one of the most common parasympathetic reflexes.)**
- Somatic dysfunction from VSR have some of the same components as SD caused by other reasons (ie, structural changes, trauma).
  - Tissue texture changes of chronic VSR—atrophied, firm, dry, cool, rubbery, ropy.
  - Tissue texture changes of acute VSR—boggy, moist, warm.
  - Restriction of motion tends to have a rubbery end feel versus the firm end feel of structural SD.
- When treated with OMT, SD of VSR origin may resolve for a short time. Unless the visceral problem is addressed, the SD will keep coming back.

When in doubt, the vagus nerve shouts.

TABLE 6-1. Viscerosomatic Reflexes

SYSTEM	SYMPATHETIC (THORACOLUMBAR)		PARASYMPATHETIC (CRANIOSACRAL)	COMMENTS
HEENT/Neck	T1-T4 bilateral		CN V, C0, C1, C2	
Cardiac	T1-T5 (left > right)		C0, C1, C2	T2 on the L is specific for an MI
Pulmonary	T1-T4 bilateral		C0, C1, C2	The "asthma reflex" is T2 L Vagal stimulation can exacerbate bronchospasm; don't treat C2 during an acute asthma attack
GI	Esophagus Stomach	T3-T6 R T5-T10 L	C0, C1, C2-up to transverse colon	Common GI pattern: C2 L, T3 R, T5 L, T7 R
	Duodenum Appendix Liver and gall bladder	T6-T8 R T9-T12 R T6-T9 R	S2-S4 (pelvic splanchnics)—transverse colon to anus	Ascending colon is right-sided; descending colon is left-sided
	Pancreas Spleen Small intestine Colon and rectum	T5-T9 bilateral T7-T9 L T8-T10 bilateral T10-L2		
GU (think thoracolumbar junction)	Kidneys	T9-L1 bilateral	C0, C1, C2	
	Ureters and bladder	T10-L2	S2-S4	
	Prostate	T10-L2	S2-S4	
	Ovaries (testes) and fallopian tubes	T9-T11	S2-S4 (for fallopian tubes)	
	Uterus and cervix	T10-L1	S2-S4	

CN, cranial nerve; GI, gastrointestinal; GU, genitourinary; HEENT, head, eyes, ears, nose and throat.

LOCATIONS OF VSRs

Table 6-1 lists the locations of specific VSR. Several sources were used to comprise this list. Keep in mind that for board purposes, VSR can be plus or minus one to two segments.

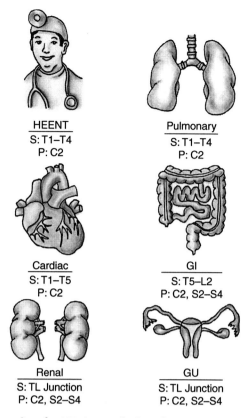

HEENT
S: T1–T4
P: C2

Pulmonary
S: T1–T4
P: C2

Cardiac
S: T1–T5
P: C2

GI
S: T5–L2
P: C2, S2–S4

Renal
S: TL Junction
P: C2, S2–S4

GU
S: TL Junction
P: C2, S2–S4

FIGURE 6-1. **Groupings for VSR (sympathetic and parasympathetic).**

▶ CHAPMAN REFLEX POINTS

Questions addressing CRP are commonly found on the boards. Like VSR, these questions are added to the end of a case scenario and measure osteopathic diagnostic skills. They are also somatic representations of visceral disease. The CRP, like VSR, should be studied regionally. Below are drawings to help you identify the regions of somatic change associated with visceral disease.

History

- Frank Chapman, a student of A.T. Still, determined these points in the 1920s.
- Anterior and posterior points were used for diagnosis and treatment, respectively.
- Today these points are used more as diagnostic indicators for dysfunction of a particular organ.

Definition

- Small points of increased tenderness and sensitivity found in the deep fascial layers that correlate with increased sympathetic tone to a particular area of the body.
- They are a type of VSR.

153

Physiology

- Increased sympathetic tone as well as blockages in the lymphatic system lead to myofascial nodules.
- These points are less specific because of the fact that one spinal segment innervates several organs, not just one.

Physical Findings

- Location: Deep in the fascia
- Palpation: Small, smooth, firm, 2 to 3 mm, "string of pearls"
- Tissue texture change (just like VSR)
- Acute reflexes: Boggy, edematous
- Chronic reflexes: Ropy, thickened, feels like a pea
- Very sensitive and very tender but does not radiate away from the specific point
- Not necessarily associated with SD

Location of Points

(See Figures 6-2 to 6-7.)

- About 50 from head to toe.
- Bilateral on anterior and posterior surface of body.
- Anterior—located about the intercostal spaces near the sternum.
  - Level of rib segment correlates with sympathetic outflow from that same segment to the corresponding viscera
- Posterior—located at the paraspinal areas near the transverse processes.
  - Points feel more like VSR.
- If an anterior point is present, the corresponding posterior point is present too.

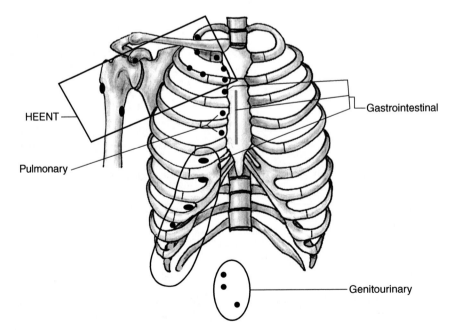

FIGURE 6-2. Anterior, upper quarter of CRP.

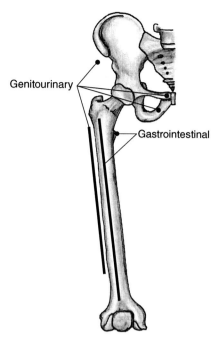

FIGURE 6-3. Anterior, lower quarter of CRP.

- Lower extremity points.
  - Located on the anterior aspect of the iliotibial band extending from just below the greater trochanter to just above the knee, bilaterally
  - Correlate to the mirror image of the abdominal contents
- If an anterior point is present, the corresponding posterior point is present too.
- Findings can help in determining a differential diagnosis (ie, visceral pathology vs. musculoskeletal pathology).

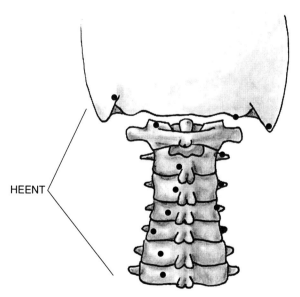

FIGURE 6-4. Posterior cervical region of CRP.

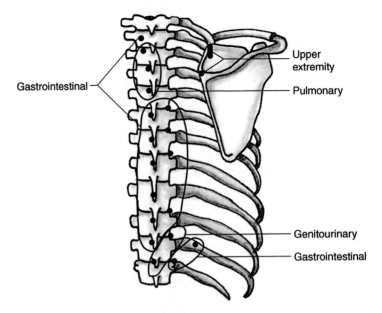

FIGURE 6-5. **Posterior thoracic region of CRP.**

Treatment

- Purpose: To decrease sympathetic tone
- Any point whether anterior or posterior may be used for diagnosis and treatment
- Technique: Contact point with pad of finger and apply a circular motion with firm pressure for 15 seconds to 2 minutes
- Release: Felt when there is a softening of tension in the fascia

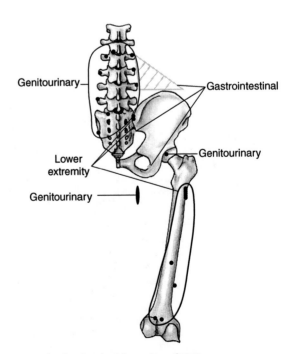

FIGURE 6-6. **Posterior lumbar/pelvis region of CRP.**

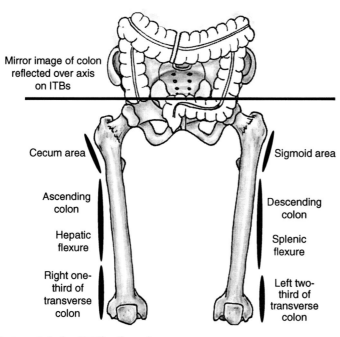

FIGURE 6-7. Anterior CRP for the colon.

Clinical Examples and Frequently Treated Points

- Appendicitis: CRP found at the tip of the right twelfth rib.
- Irritable bowel syndrome: CRP found along the iliotibial band.

▶ JONES' CS TENDERPOINTS

Jones' CS tenderpoints are the points that are used for the indirect technique of CS. Table 6-2 and Figures 6-8 through 6-15 illustrate the location of these points. As always, do not memorize every single point but rather the generalizations for each area of the body. The points found within the axial skeleton tend to be higher yield than the extremity points.

History

- Dr Lawrence H. Jones, DO, determined these points in 1955.
- His paper titled *Spontaneous Release of Positioning* was published in 1964.

Definition

- An area of tenderness or hypersensitivity that has a direct relationship to SD of an adjacent area.
- Based on the neuromuscular basis of SD.

Physiology

- An inappropriate amount of proprioceptive activity to a given area leading to a reflex tenderpoint and subsequent SD

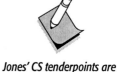

Jones' CS tenderpoints are directly related to SD.

TABLE 6-2. Location of Jones Tenderpoints; Not All-Inclusive

AREA		ANTERIOR POINTS	POSTERIOR POINTS	COMMENTS
Cervical spine (C2-C6)		Anterior surface of transverse processes of vertebrae; not on the SCM but SCM crosses this line of these points	On either side of the spinous process of the vertebral segment above the segment with SD	
Thoracic spine	T1	Apex of sternal notch	T1-T12—inferolateral aspect of spinous process of vertebra, bilaterally	The anterior points from T1 to T6 are all midline; T7-T12 are all bilateral
	T2	Middle of manubrium		
	T3-T6	On sternum at rib level		
	T7	Under costochondral margin, lateral and inferior to xiphoid		
	T8	3 cm below xiphoid		
	T9	1-2 cm above umbilicus, 2-3 cm lateral to midline		
	T10	1-2 cm below umbilicus laterally		
	T11	5-6 cm below umbilicus and laterally		
	T12	Inner surface of iliac crest at mid-axillary line		
Ribs	R1	At point of articulation with manubrium	R2-R6—posterior aspect of ribs at rib angles	
	R2	Second rib mid-clavicular		
	R3-R6	On rib at anterior axillary line		
	R7-R12	Uncommon		
Lumbar	L1	Medial side of ASIS	L1-L5—inferolateral side of spinous process, bilaterally; can also be midline directly on the spinous process	
	L2	Medial side of AIIS		
	L3	Lateral side of AIIS		
	L4	Inferior side of AIIS		
	L5	Pubic rami, 1 cm lateral to pubic symphysis		
Pelvis				
Iliacus		Halfway between the midline and the ASIS at the level of the ilium		
Lower pole fifth lumbar		2 cm below PSIS of ilium		
Piriformis		Within the muscle belly, half way between the attachments (greater trochanter and anterior aspect of ILA of sacrum)		

AREA	ANTERIOR POINTS	POSTERIOR POINTS	COMMENTS
Extremities			
Supraspinatus	Within the muscle belly		
Subscapularis	Anterolateral surface of scapula		
Biceps brachii	Tendon of long head of biceps in the bicipital groove		
Rectus femoris	Musculotendinous region at distal end, above patella		
Gastrocnemius	Muscle bellies of both heads of the muscle		

AIIS, anterior inferior iliac spine; ASIS, anterior superior iliac spine; ILA, inferior lateral angle; PSIS, posterior superior iliac spine; SCM, sternocleidomastoid.

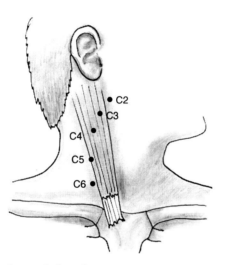

FIGURE 6-8. Anterior cervical tenderpoints.

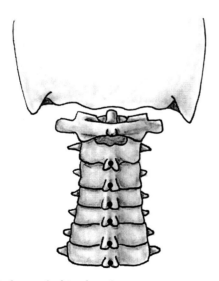

FIGURE 6-9. Posterior cervical tenderpoints.

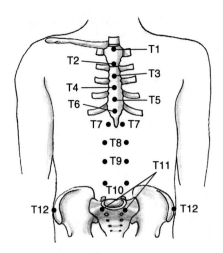

FIGURE 6-10. Anterior thoracic tenderpoints.

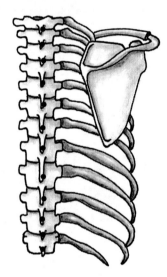

FIGURE 6-11. Posterior thoracic tenderpoints.

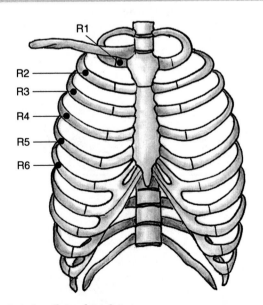

FIGURE 6-12. Anterior rib tenderpoints.

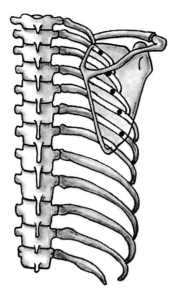

FIGURE 6-13. Posterior rib tenderpoints.

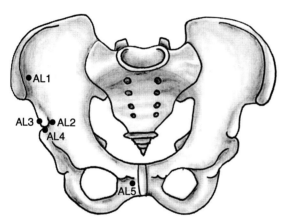

FIGURE 6-14. Anterior lumbar tenderpoints.

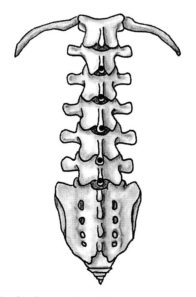

FIGURE 6-15. Posterior lumbar tenderpoints.

Physical Findings

- Tense, fibrotic, dime-sized
- The amount of tenderness perceived by the patient is inappropriate for the amount of pressure being used by the examiner.
- Location of tenderpoints is consistent from one person to the next.
- Similar to CRP in that the pain doesn't radiate.

Location of Points

(See Table 6-2.)

Treatment

- The body is placed into a position of maximum comfort.
- Tenderness on the point should be reduced by approximately two-thirds.
- The position of comfort is almost always held for 90 seconds.
- The patient remains passive as the physician returns them to a neutral position.

> ▶ **MUSCULOSKELETAL TESTS**

Musculoskeletal medicine and osteopathic manipulative medicine (OMM) are integrated throughout the COMLEX. Common orthopedic tests used in specific musculoskeletal medicine situations are reviewed in the following table.

Common Upper and Lower Extremity Musculoskeletal Tests

Region	Name of Test	Description	+ Findings
Neck	Adson test (Figure 6-16)	The radial pulse is palpated and the patient is directed to rotate and extend the head away from the side of the complaint. The patient inhales and holds the breath. This is repeated again with the patient rotating and extending the head toward the side of the complaint	The radial pulse decreases or disappears; **indicates thoracic outlet syndrome**
	Spurling test (Figures 6-17 A and B)	A compressive force is transmitted down the axial spine through the top of the head. Compression is given with the neck in neutral, sidebent left, and sidebent right	Patient will have radiating symptoms down the arms into the hands; **indicates a cervical nerve root impingement**
Shoulder	Apley scratch test (Figures 6-18 A and B)	Patient reaches behind back to touch opposite shoulder blade. Patient reaches above and behind head to ward the shoulder blades	Determines **ranges of motion of internal rotation, abduction, and adduction.** If these motions are limited, there will be asymmetry from one side to the other

Common Upper and Lower Extremity Musculoskeletal Tests (Continued)

Region	Name of Test	Description	+ Findings
	Apprehension/ Relocation test (Figures 6-19 A and B)	With the elbow flexed to 90° and the humerus abducted to 90°, the GH joint is brought into passive external rotation	Pain is elicited and the patient becomes apprehensive with increased external rotation. When **relocated** by stabilizing the humeral head, the patient gets relief; **indicates anterior GH laxity**
	Empty can test (Jobe test) (Figure 6-20)	The GH joint is abducted to 90°, horizontally flexed to 30°, and internally rotated 90° (thumb points downward). The patient resists a downward force exerted at the forearm by the examiner, while the examiner stabilizes the GH joint	One arm will demonstrate an inability to resist the downward force and may drop more quickly than the other arm. Pain is also elicited at the greater tuberosity of the humerus; **indicates a supraspinatus tendonitis or tear**
	Hawkins-Kennedy impingement test (Figure 6-21)	The GH joint is at 90° of abduction and 30° of forward flexion; the elbow is flexed to 90°; the humerus is then internally rotated	Pain; **indicates impingement of the rotator cuff tendons (usually supraspinatus)**
	Neer sign (Figure 6-22)	With the elbow extended and the GH joint internally rotated, the GH joint is passively brought into full forward flexion	Pain; **indicates impingement of the rotator cuff tendons (usually supraspinatus)**
	Speed test (Figure 6-23)	The elbow is extended with the palm facing up. The patient resists flexion of the GH joint	Pain occurs with resisted flexion; **indicates tendonitis of the long head of the biceps or a possible labral injury**
	Sulcus sign (Figure 6-24)	While holding the patient's arm at the elbow, downward traction is applied by the examiner	A sulcus (depression) appears below the glenoid; **indicates inferior GH laxity**

Region	Name of Test	Description	+ Findings
	Yergason test (Figure 6-25)	The elbow is flexed to 90° and the patient resists while the examiner brings the GH joint into external rotation and pulls the elbow inferiorly	Popping or snapping at the bicipital groove; **indicates laxity of the transverse humeral ligament. Pain without popping or snapping indicates bicipital tendonitis**
Elbow, wrist, hand	Finkelstein test (Figure 6-26)	The patient makes a fist, tucking the thumb inside the fingers; the wrist is actively moved into ulnar deviation	Pain on the radial side; **indicates tenosynovitis of the extensor pollicis brevis and abductor pollicis longus tendons (de Quervain syndrome/ tenosynovitis)**
	Phalen test (Figures 6-27 A and B)	Patient places the dorsal aspect of both wrists together causing excessive flexion at the wrists. The position is held for 1 minute	Tingling will occur in the distribution of the median nerve (lateral three and a half digits); **indicates carpal tunnel.** Reverse Phalen (placing palmar aspect together) will alleviate symptoms
	Tinel sign (Figure 6-28)	Tapping over the median nerve at the transverse carpal ligament	Pain and tingling radiating into the fingers of the distribution of the median nerve; **indicates carpal tunnel**
Lower back, hips, SI	FABERE sign (Patrick test) (Figure 6-29)	The patient is lying supine with the foot of the involved side resting on the opposite thigh. This position brings the hip into flexion, abduction, external rotation, and extension. The examiner stabilizes the opposite ASIS while pushing downward on the knee of the involved side	Pain in the SI joint **indicates SI pathology.** Pain in the anterior aspect of the femur indicates hip pathology

Region	Name of Test	Description	+ Findings
	Iliac compression/ distraction test (Figures 6-30 A and B)	The patient is lying supine. The examiner exerts a force laterally at the ASIS bilaterally which causes compression of the SI joints. The examiner then exerts a force medially at the ilium bilaterally which causes gapping of the SI joints	Pain with compression of the SI joints and relief of pain with spreading of the SI joints; **indicates SI pathology**
	Backward bending test (single leg stance test) (Figure 6-31)	While standing, the patient lifts one leg and extends at the waist. This same motion is repeated while standing on the opposite side	Pain in the lumbar spine area; **indicates pathology of a posterior element (ie, spondylolysis, spondylolisthesis, or facet DJD)**
	Straight leg raise test (Figure 6-32)	The patient is lying supine with the involved leg extended. The examiner grasps the heel with one hand while keeping the knee in full extension with the other hand. The examiner begins to lift the leg causing flexion of the hip	Pain, paresthesias radiating down the leg between 30° and 70° of hip flexion; **indicates irritation of the sciatic nerve or lumbar nerve root.** Pathology could stem from a bulging/ herniated disc *or* piriformis syndrome where the tightened piriformis is clamping down on the sciatic nerve leading to symptoms
	Thomas test (Figures 6-33 A and B)	The patient is lying supine with the buttocks at the end of the table; one knee is drawn up to the chest while the other leg (the one being tested) remains passive	The **knee** of the tested leg is unable to flex to 90°; **indicates a tight rectus femoris.** The **thigh** of the tested leg raises off the table; **indicates a tight iliopsoas**
	Trendelenburg test (Figures 6-34 A and B)	While standing, the patient raises the leg opposite the side being tested	The iliac crest of the non–weight-bearing side falls below the level of the iliac crest on the standing leg; **indicates weakness of the gluteus medius of the standing leg**

Region	Name of Test	Description	+ Findings
	Valsalva test (Figure 6-35)	While seated, the patient bears down on a closed glottis causing an increase in intrathecal pressure	Pain in the spine; **indicates a herniated disc at the level of the pain**
Knee	Anterior drawer test (Figure 6-36)	The patient is lying supine with the hip flexed to 45° and the knee to 90°. The examiner sits on the foot of the patient to fix the distal tibia. The proximal tibia is pulled forward by grasping the lower leg posteriorly, just below the joint line of the knee. This should be done with the hip in neutral, at 20° of internal rotation, and at 15° to 20° of external rotation	Increased anterior tibial translation when compared to the opposite side; **indicates a tear of the ACL**
	Apley compression test (Figure 6-37)	The patient is lying prone with the knee flexed to 90°. The examiner contacts the calcaneus and exerts an axial load through the tibia while simultaneously introducing internal rotation and then external rotation	Joint line pain with compression; **indicates a tear of the meniscus and or collateral ligaments**
	Apley distraction test (Figure 6-38)	The patient is lying prone with the knee flexed to 90°. The examiner grasps the ankle with one hand while stabilizing the femur on the table with the other. A distraction force is applied through the ankle to affect the knee while simultaneously introducing internal and external rotation	Pain with distraction; consistent with a **tear of the collateral ligaments.** Alleviation of pain following Apley compression is indicative of **meniscal pathology**
	Lachman test (Figure 6-39)	The patient is lying supine with the knee passively flexed to 20°. The examiner grasps the tibia with one hand and stabilizes the femur with the other hand. The tibia is anteriorly translated while the femur is pushed posteriorly	Increased anterior tibial translation when compared to the opposite side; **indicates a tear of the ACL**
	McMurray test (Figures 6-40 A and B)	The patient is lying supine. The examiner monitors the joint line with one hand while holding the patient's distal tibia with the other. The examiner passively flexes the knee while simultaneously internally and externally rotating the tibia. A gentle valgus stress is then placed on the knee with the tibia externally rotated while the knee is slowly and passively extended	Popping, clicking, or locking of the knee and pain in the joint line; **indicates a tear of the meniscus (either medial, lateral, or both, depending on location of symptoms—usually medial)**

Region	Name of Test	Description	+ Findings
	Ober test (Figures 6-41 A and B)	The patient is sidelying with the affected side up and both knees and hips flexed to 90°. The examiner stabilizes the pelvis with one hand while lifting and extending the affected hip and returning it to neutral. The hip is then allowed to drop (adduct) to the table	The knee does not drop to the table; **indicates an ITB**
	Posterior drawer test (Figure 6-42)	The patient and examiner are set up in the exact same way as with the Anterior drawer test. The tibia is pushed posteriorly	Increased posterior tibial translation when compared to the opposite side; **indicates a tear of the PCL**
	Valgus stress test (Figure 6-43)	The patient is lying supine. The examiner grasps the distal tibia with one hand while exerting a valgus (medial) force with the other hand at the level of the joint line of the knee, performed at complete extension and at 20° to 30° of knee	Increased laxity at the medial knee when compared to the opposite side; **indicates a tear of the MCL**
	Varus stress test (Figure 6-44)	The patient is lying supine. The examiner stands between the table and the leg. The examiner grasps the distal tibia with one hand while exerting a varus (lateral) force with the other hand at the level of the joint line of the knee, performed at complete extension and at 20° to 30° of knee flexion	Increased laxity at the lateral knee when compared to the opposite side; **indicates a tear of the LCL**
Lower leg, ankle, foot	Anterior drawer test (Figure 6-45)	With the lower leg dangling off the table and the foot in slight plantar flexion, the examiner pulls the calcaneus and talus forward while stabilizing the a distal tibia	Increased laxity compared to the other side, pain, or clunk; **indicates a tear of the ATF ligament. This is the most commonly injured ligament in ankle sprains**
	Bump test (Figure 6-46)	The patient is seated with the foot off the table. The examiner uses the palm of the hand to bump the calcaneus with increasing force	Pain in the area of the calcaneus, talus, tibia or fibula; **indicates an advanced stress fracture**

Region	Name of Test	Description	+ Findings
	Kleiger test (Figure 6-47)	With the lower leg dangling off the table, the foot is rotated laterally (not inverted or everted) while the tibia is stabilized	Pain on the medial aspect; **indicates a sprain of the deltoid ligament.** Pain superior to the lateral malleolus; **indicates a sprain of the syndesmosis**
	Squeeze test (Figure 6-48)	The examiner squeezes the proximal tibia and fibula together with increasing pressure	Pain in the distal leg; **indicates a fracture of the tibia, fibula, or a sprain of the syndesmosis**
	Thompson test (Simmonds test) (Figure 6-49)	With the patient prone or seated with the foot off the table, the examiner squeezes the calf	No plantar flexion of the foot; **indicates a tear of the Achilles tendon**
	Talar tilt test (inversion/ eversion stress test) (Figures 6-50 A and B)	With the lower leg dangling off the table, the examiner grasps the calcaneus and brings it into inversion and eversion	Increased tilting compared to the other side; **indicates a sprain of the CF ligament and the deltoid ligament, respectively**

ACL, anterior cruciate ligament; ASIS, anterior superior iliac spine; ATF, anterior talofibular (ligament); CF, calcaneofibular; DJD, degenerative joint disease; GH, glenohumeral; ITB, iliotibial band; LCL, lateral collateral ligament; MCL, medial collateral ligament; PCL, posterior cruciate ligament; SI, sacroiliac.

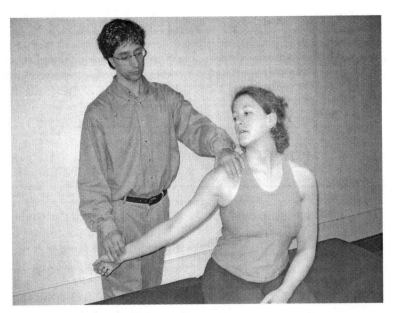

FIGURE 6-16. Adson test.

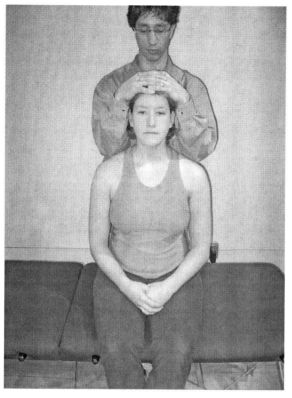

FIGURE 6-17(A). Spurling test in neutral.

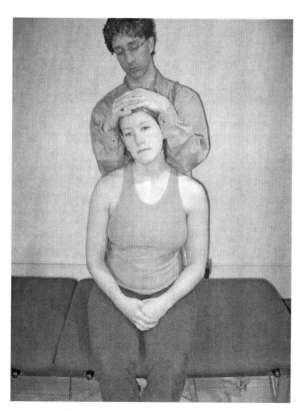

FIGURE 6-17(B). Spurling test with neck sidebent to one side.

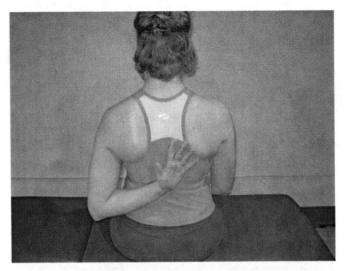

FIGURE 6-18(A). Apley scratch test. Testing internal rotation and adduction.

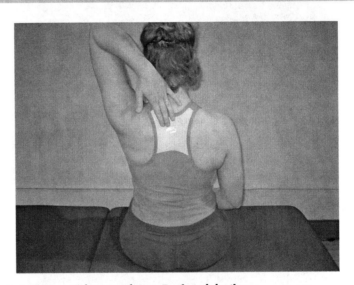

FIGURE 6-18(B). Apley scratch test. Testing abduction.

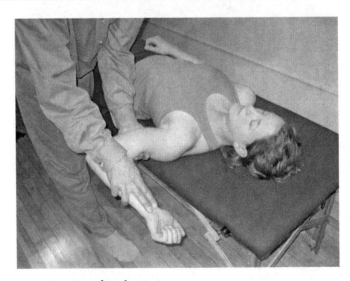

FIGURE 6-19(A). Apprehension test.

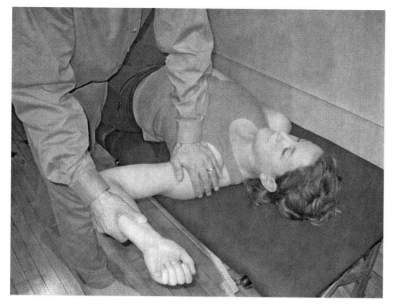

FIGURE 6-19(B). Relocation test.

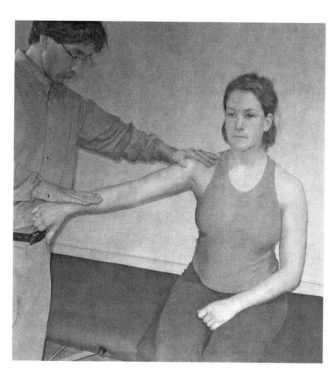

FIGURE 6-20. Jobe/Empty can test.

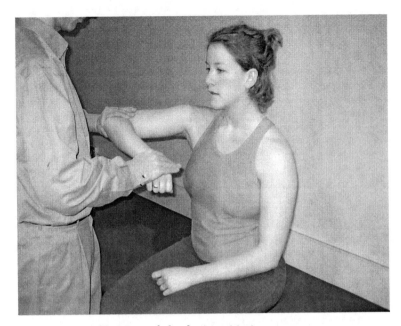

FIGURE 6-21. Hawkins-Kennedy impingement test.

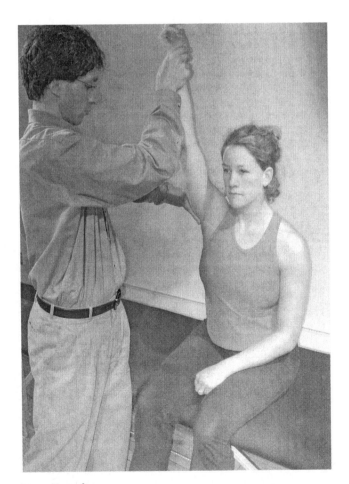

FIGURE 6-22. Neer sign.

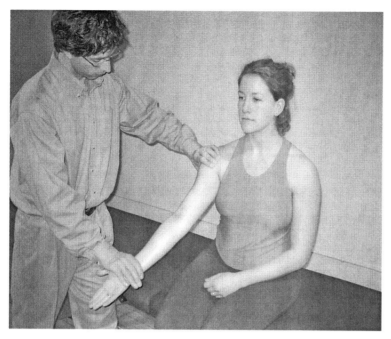

FIGURE 6-23. Speed test.

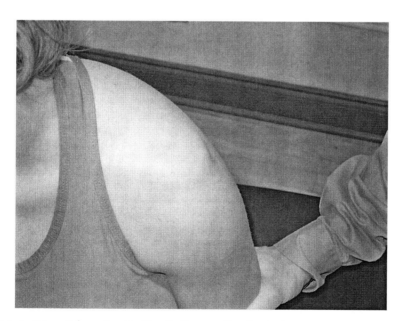

FIGURE 6-24. Sulcus sign. Positive findings; notice depression.

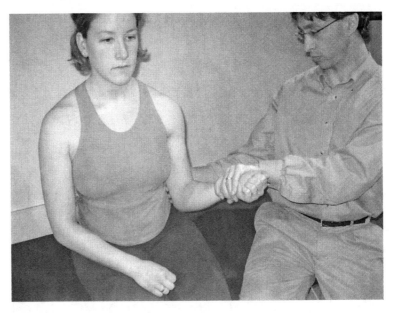

FIGURE 6-25. Yergason test.

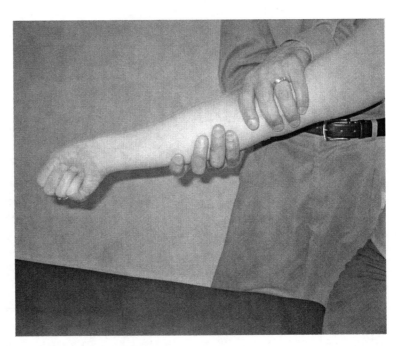

FIGURE 6-26. Finkelstein test.

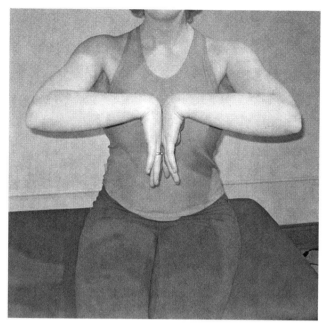

FIGURE 6-27(A).   Phalen test.

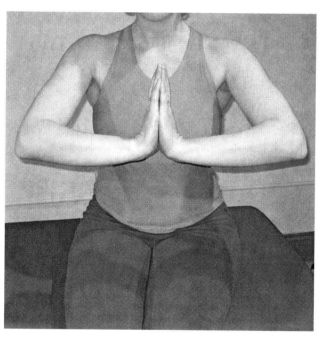

FIGURE 6-27(B).   Reverse Phalen test.

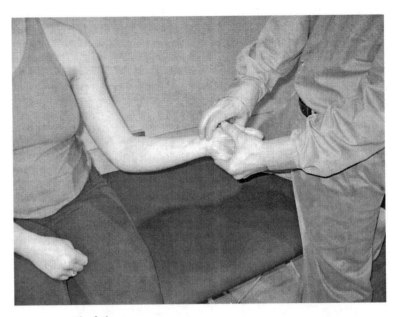

FIGURE 6-28. Tinel sign.

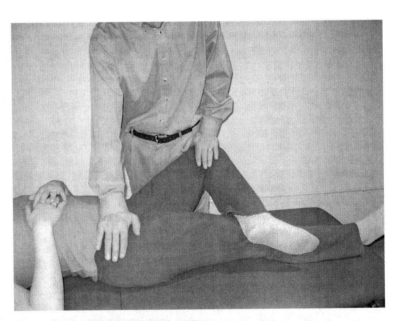

FIGURE 6-29. FABERE sign (Patrick test).

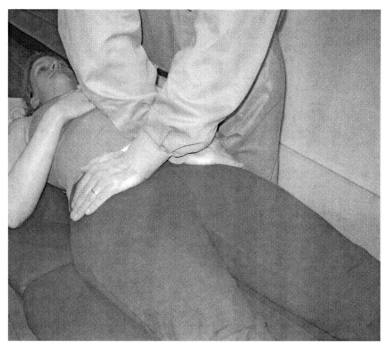

FIGURE 6-30(A). Iliac compression test.

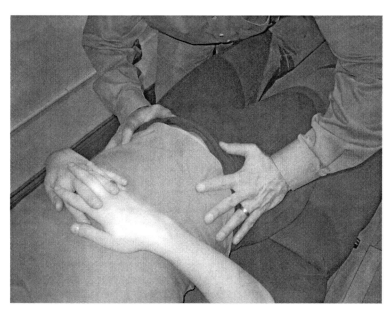

FIGURE 6-30(B). Iliac distraction test.

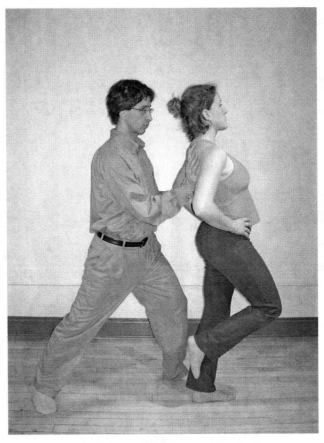

FIGURE 6-31. Backward bending test (single leg stance test).

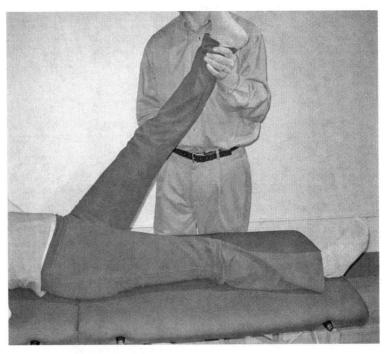

FIGURE 6-32. Straight leg raise test.

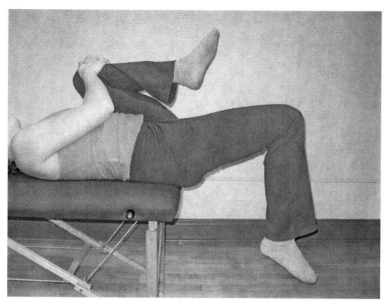

FIGURE 6-33(A).   Thomas test. Positive for tight rectus femoris.

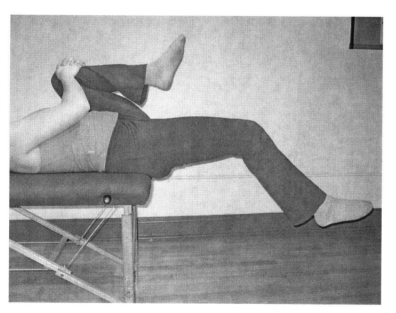

FIGURE 6-33(B).   Thomas test. Positive for tight iliopsoas.

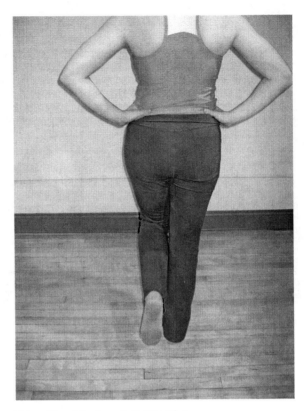

FIGURE 6-34(A). Trendelenburg test. Negative.

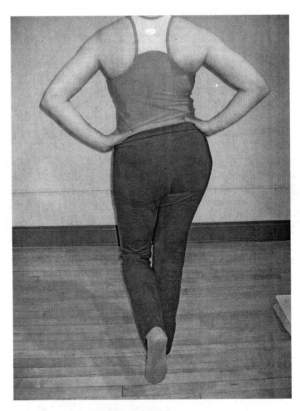

FIGURE 6-34(B). Trendelenburg test. Positive.

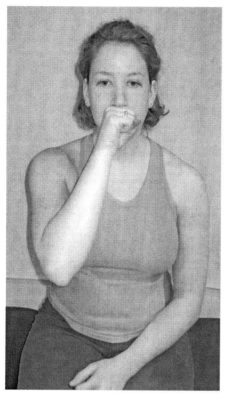

FIGURE 6-35. Valsalva test.

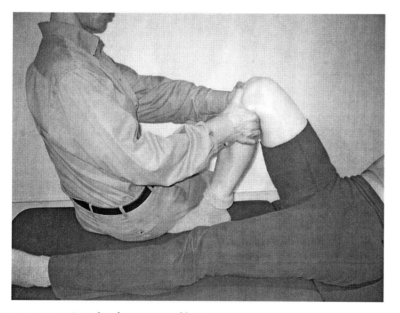

FIGURE 6-36. Anterior drawer test of knee.

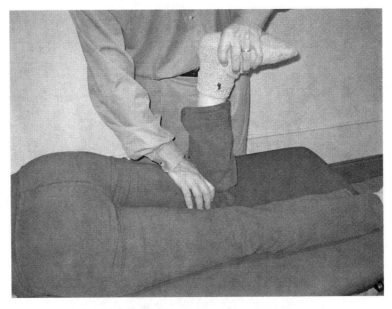

FIGURE 6-37. Apley compression test.

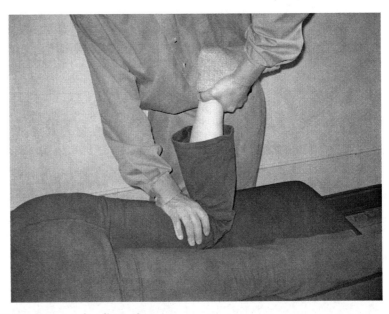

FIGURE 6-38. Apley distraction test.

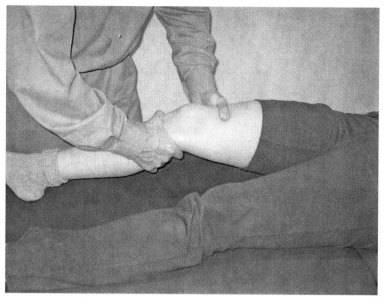

FIGURE 6-39. Lachman test.

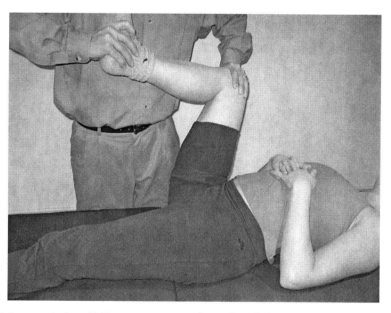

FIGURE 6-40(A). McMurray test. External rotation of tibia.

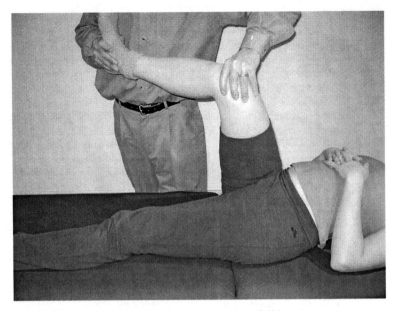

FIGURE 6-40(B). McMurray test. Internal rotation of tibia.

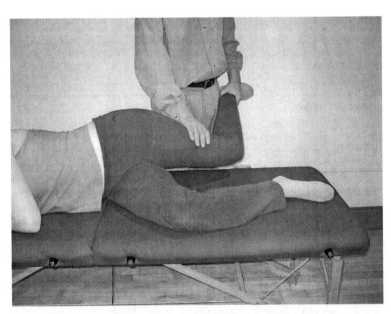

FIGURE 6-41(A). Ober test. Negative; knee falls onto table.

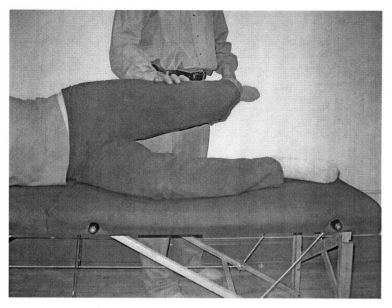

FIGURE 6-41(B). Ober test. Positive.

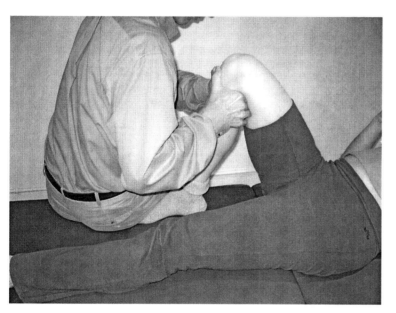

FIGURE 6-42. Posterior drawer test.

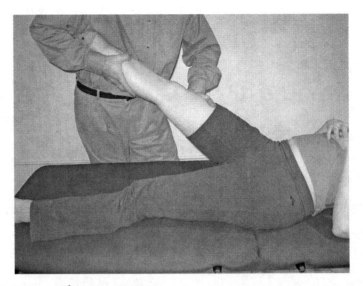

FIGURE 6-43. Valgus stress test.

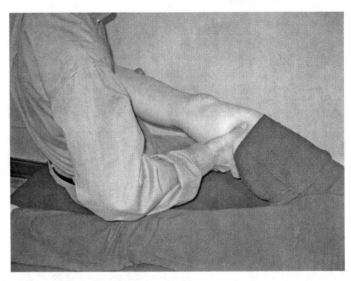

FIGURE 6-44. Varus stress test.

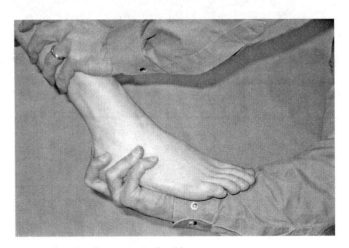

FIGURE 6-45. Anterior drawer test of ankle.

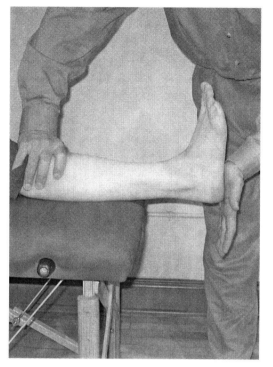

FIGURE 6-46. Bump test.

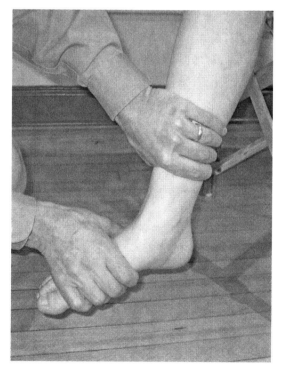

FIGURE 6-47. Kleiger test.

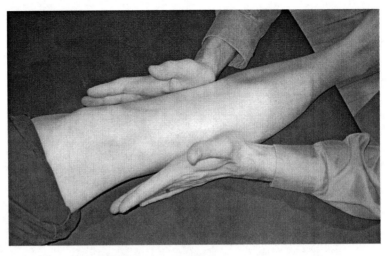

FIGURE 6-48. Squeeze test.

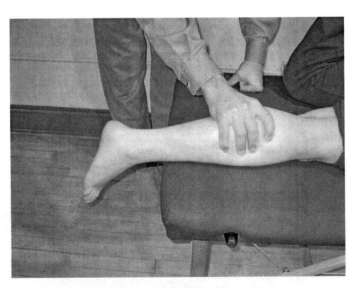

FIGURE 6-49. Thompson test (Simmonds test).

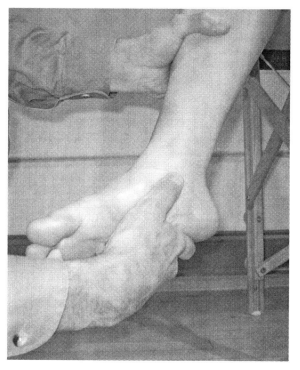

FIGURE 6-50(A). Talar tilt test (inversion).

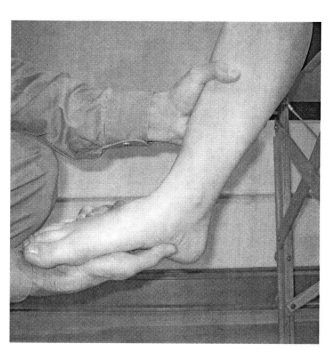

FIGURE 6-50(B). Talar tilt test (eversion).

Osteopathic Treatments and Techniques

Cranial Treatment

Vault Contact

(See Figure 7-1.)

INDICATIONS

- Used to diagnose cranial strain patterns.
- Patient is in supine position.
- Commonly used to count cranial rhythmic impulse (CRI), observe flexion and extension of sphenobasilar synchondrosis (SBS).

TECHNIQUE

> *Remember, the SBS rises in cranial flexion and falls in cranial extension.*

- Index fingers are placed in area of the greater wings of the sphenoid.
- Middle fingers are placed on the temporal bones anterior to the external auditory meatus.
- Ring fingers are placed on the temporal bones posterior to the external auditory meatus, above the mastoid process.
- Fifth fingers are placed near lateral angle of occiput.
- From this hold, it may be convenient to diagnose cranial strain patterns.

Anteroposterior Contact

(See Figure 7-2.)

- Can be used seated or supine.
- The operator sits at the side of table.
- The operator's posterior hand is placed under patient's head such that physician's palm contacts the squamous portion of occiput.

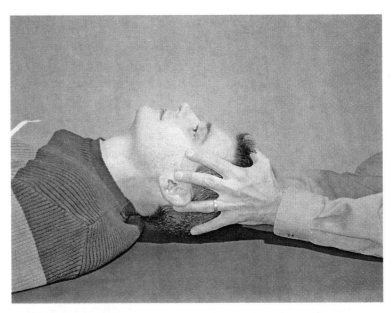

FIGURE 7-1. Vault contact.

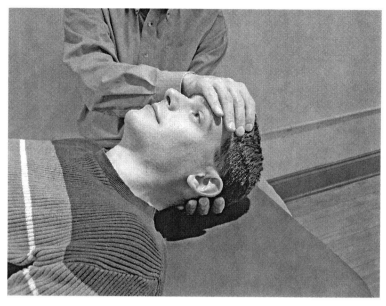

FIGURE 7-2. AP contact.

- The physician's thumbs are pointed toward the patient's head.
- Superior hand contacts sphenoid such that the physician's thumb is in the area of the greater wing and the fourth and fifth digits are across the forehead contacting the opposite greater wing of sphenoid.
- This contact allows appreciation of dural membrane motion as well as bony articular motion.

Sacral Contact

- Can be palpated either supine or prone position

PATIENT PRONE

- The base of physician's hand is placed in area of base of the patient's sacrum. The other hand is placed on top of the palpating hand.

PATIENT SUPINE 1

(See Figure 7-3.)

- The physician sits at the side of the table facing the head of the patient.
- The patient's hips and knees are flexed. Physician's hand is placed in the area of the patient's sacrum such that the operator's fingertips are inferior to L5.
- The physician's hand, wrist, and forearm should all be straight, with minimal weight placed on the physician's elbow.

PATIENT SUPINE 2

(See Figure 7-4.)

- Physician sits at the side of the table, facing the head of the patient.
- The patient rolls toward the operator, while the physician's hand is placed between the patient's legs, contacting the sacrum.

Remember, the sacral base moves posteriorly and superiorly with cranial flexion, and anteriorly and inferiorly with cranial extension.

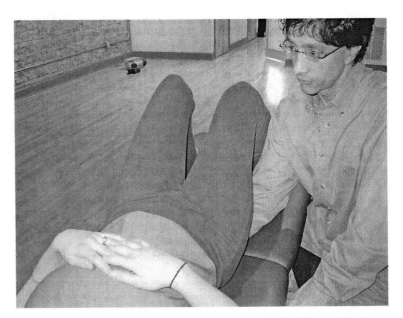

FIGURE 7-3. Sacral hold 1.

- The patient is then instructed to return to supine position. Again, the physician's hand, wrist, and forearm should all be straight, with minimal weight placed on the table.
- For infants or obese patients, the patient can be supine while the physician uses two fingers in a "V" position to palpate the sacrum. In larger patients, the physician can palpate the sacrococcygeal angle.
- The sacrum follows the occiput; therefore, one can palpate the reciprocal tension membrane (RTM) via the sacrum.

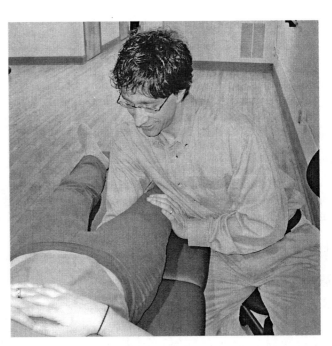

FIGURE 7-4. Sacral hold 2.

V-Spread Technique

INDICATIONS

- Used for compression of any suture, but often used for the occipitomastoid suture.
- Ninety percent of the venous drainage from the head occurs through the internal jugular vein, which courses through the jugular foramen in close proximity to the occipitomastoid suture.
- Compression of the occipitomastoid suture can reduce drainage from the head and affect cranial nerves IX to XI via the jugular foramen.
- Useful for any pathology associated with the above nerves.

CV4 Technique

INDICATIONS

- Used to stimulate the inherent therapeutic force of the body by compressing the fourth ventricle
- Useful for increasing overall motion, rate, and amplitude
- Useful for achieving a balanced autonomic nervous system

Frontal and Parietal Lift

INDICATIONS

- Lifts are used to balance membranous tension.
- Frontal lift is particularly useful in treating sinus dysfunction.

On boards, often the treatment of choice when patient is described as having low rate and amplitude of the CRI

CHAPTER 8

Cervical Treatment

High Velocity, Low Amplitude: Occiput Posterior (flexed)

(See Figure 8-1.)

- With the patient supine and the physician at the head of the table, the physician contacts the posterior (flexed) occipital condyle with the metacarpophalangeal (MCP) joint of their index finger. The physician's opposite hand cradles the patient's head while introducing sidebending to the side of the dysfunction.
- The physician applies a force through the MCP joint of their index finger through the posterior (flexed) occipital condyle, inducing rotation away from the dysfunction.
- When the restrictive barrier is reached, the corrective force is with the MCP joint through the posterior (flexed) occipital condyle causing further rotation.
- Reassess.

Muscle Energy: Occiput Posterior (flexed)

- The same position as above is achieved.
- When the restrictive barrier is reached, the physician asks the patient to rotate their head against resistance of the physician's hold. This is held for 3 to 5 seconds and then released. After waiting for 3 seconds, the physician introduces further rotation to engage the new restrictive barrier.
- Repeat three to four times, until normal range of motion is restored to the occiput on the atlas.
- Reassess.

Indirect: Occiput Posterior (flexed)

- With the patient lying supine and the physician at the head of the table, the physician contacts the nondysfunctional occipital condyle with the

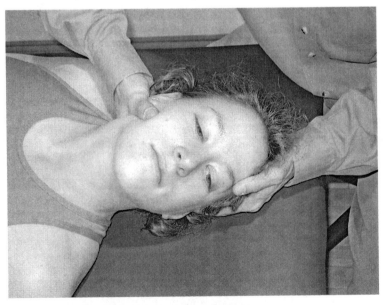

FIGURE 8-1. HVLA–occiput posterior left (flexed left).

MCP joint of their index finger. With the pads of their opposite index and middle fingertips, contact the dysfunctional occipital condyle.

▪ The physician applies a force through the MCP joint of their hand contacting the nondysfunctional occipital condyle, inducing rotation toward the dysfunction. With the opposite hand, he/she applies about 10% of the force by pulling the posterior (flexed) occipital condyle further posteriorly, assisting rotation of the occiput.

▪ This position is held until a release is felt.

▪ Reassess.

High Velocity, Low Amplitude: Posterior Atlas

(See Figure 8-2.)

▪ With the patient supine and physician at the head of the table, the physician places the MCP joint against the posterior aspect of the atlas (the lateral mass). The opposite hand is placed on the parietal bone of the cranium.

▪ The physician applies pressure with their hand against the posterior aspect of the atlas on the dysfunctional side and rotates the head away from the dysfunction. The opposite hand is used as a support to guide the head.

▪ The head is rotated, until the restrictive barrier is met. At this point, a quick thrust through the physician's hand is applied to rotate the patient's atlas further into the restrictive barrier. The patient's head is then brought back to neutral.

▪ Reassess the rotation of the atlas on the axis.

> *Remember, the dysfunction of the atlas is in its major motion: rotation.*

Muscle Energy: Posterior Atlas

▪ With the patient supine and physician at the head of the table, the physician places the MCP joint of their index finger contacting the posterior aspect of the atlas (the lateral mass). The opposite hand is placed on the parietal bone of the cranium.

▪ The physician applies pressure with their hand to rotate the atlas into the restrictive barrier. The opposite hand is used as a support to guide the head.

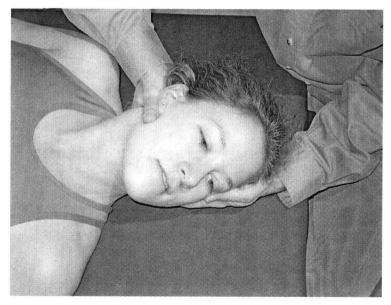

FIGURE 8-2. HVLA–dysfunction posterior left atlas.

- The head is rotated, until the restrictive barrier is met. At this point, the patient is asked to rotate their head away from the restrictive barrier. This is held for 3 to 5 seconds and then released. After waiting for 3 seconds, the physician introduces further rotation to engage the new restrictive barrier.
- This is repeated three to four times, until normal range of motion is restored.
- Reassess.

Indirect: Posterior Atlas

- With the patient supine and physician at the head of the table, the physician places the pad of their index finger on the posterior aspect of atlas (lateral mass). The pad of their opposite index finger is on the anterior aspect of the atlas (opposite lateral mass). The palms of each hand lie on the respective parietal bones of the cranium.
- The physician rotates the head of the patient away from the restrictive barrier until a balance point is reached.
- This position is held, until a release is felt.
- Reassess.

Facilitated Positional Release: Posterior Atlas

(See Figure 8-3.)

Remember, FPR is an indirect technique that utilizes a facilitating force.

- The same position of the physician and the patient is achieved as above; however, a compression force is applied through the head down the spine to the level of the atlas, then the indirect positioning of the head is achieved.
- Release is typically achieved in about 3 to 5 seconds.
- Reassess.

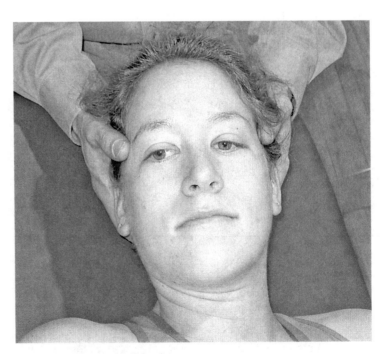

FIGURE 8-3. FPR–posterior left atlas.

High Velocity, Low Amplitude: Dysfunction: C4FRS$_R$

(See Figure 8-4.)

- With the patient lying supine and physician at the head of the table, the physician places their right hand under the patient's neck. The metacarpophalangeal (MCP) joint of the physician's right index finger contacts the posterior aspect of C4 (the right lateral mass). The patient's head is allowed to fall posteriorly and rest on the table over the physician's right hand. This allows for the extension of C4. The physician's right thumb will be resting on the patient's right cheek, pointing toward the patient's right eye. The physician's left hand contacts the patient's forehead, with the palm of their left hand contacting the frontal bone, fingers pointing to the left.
- The physician applies a force upward toward the patient's eyes at a 45° angle, through their right MCP joint of their right index finger into the right lateral mass, causing rotation left. The left hand guides this motion. The patient's head remains on the table to ensure left sidebending.
- When the restrictive barrier is met, the final force is a gentle thrust upward and to the left, at a 45° angle through the patient's eyes.
- Return to neutral position.
- Reassess.

Muscle Energy: Dysfunction C4FRS$_R$

- The same position as above is achieved.
- With the patient's head rotated and sidebent left, the physician asks the patient to gently return their head to a neutral position.
- This is held for 3 to 5 seconds and then released.
- After waiting for 3 seconds, the physician introduces further right rotation to engage the new restrictive barrier.
- Step 2 is repeated three to four times.
- Reassess.

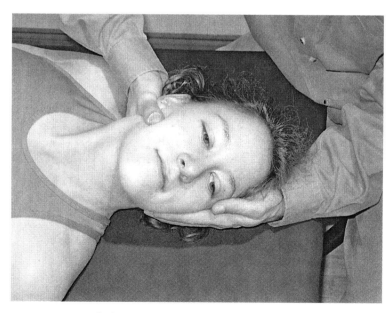

FIGURE 8-4. HVLA–dysfunction: C4FRS$_R$.

Indirect: Dysfunction C4FRS$_R$

- With the patient lying supine and physician at the head of the table, the physician places the pad of their right index finger on the posterior aspect of C4 (lateral mass). The pad of the left index finger is on the opposite lateral mass. The palms of each hand lie on the respective parietal bones of the cranium.
- The physician slowly flexes the patient's head until flexion at the level of C4 is achieved, straightening the cervical lordosis.
- The physician laterally translates their right index finger to the left causing sidebending right.
- The physician applies a superior force with their left index finger to the left lateral mass causing right rotation of the vertebra.
- This position is held until a release is felt.
- Reassess.

Facilitated Positional Release: Dysfunction C4FRS$_R$

- The same position of the physician and patient is achieved as above; however, a compression force is applied through the head down the spine to the level of C4, once indirect positioning of the vertebra is achieved.
- This position is held until a release is felt.
- Reassess.

CHAPTER 9

Thoracic, Rib, and Diaphragm Techniques

ME for Thoracic Curve, Convex Left, T3 to T7

(See Figure 9-1.)

The apex of this curve is at T5 so this will be the focus of the treatment. T5 is rotated left, sidebent right.

- Patient seated, physician standing on side of concavity.
- Physician palpates the interspinous space of T5–T6 with middle finger. Other fingers are placed in the interspinous spinous above and below this.
- Physician flexes patient's trunk minimally until gapping is felt at the T5–T6 space.
- Physician then rotates and sidebends patient's trunk into the "featheredge" of the barrier, rotating right and sidebending left.
- Patient is instructed to counteract these forces for 3 to 5 seconds.
- Forces are gently relaxed. Wait 3 to 5 seconds, and engage new barrier.
- Repeat three to five times.

HVLA (Kirksville crunch) for T4 Extended, Rotated Right, Sidebent Right—T4ER$_R$S$_R$

(See Figure 9-2.)

- Patient supine with arms hugging upper chest. Physician on side opposite of the lesion.
- Physician cradles patient's head and neck with right arm, while left thenar eminence is placed under the transverse process of T4. The physician's epigastrium is placed over the patient's elbows. A pillow can be placed over the patient's elbows for the physician's comfort.
- Patient's head and neck are flexed to T4 to T5. Left sidebending is induced from above. A small amount of left rotation can be induced to localize all planes to the barrier.

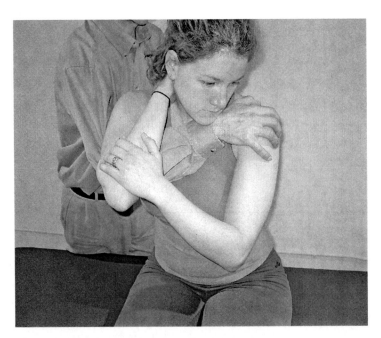

FIGURE 9-1. Muscle energy treatment of a group curve.

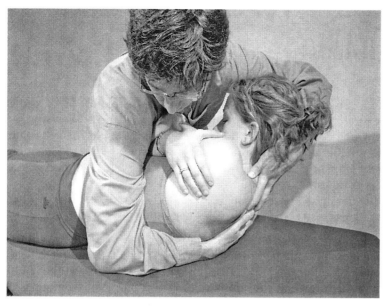

FIGURE 9-2. Kirksville crunch of a segmental dysfunction.

⬚ Final corrective force is a quick thrust through the epigastric contact in the direction of the posterior component, T4.
⬚ Note: this is one version of the technique and is the version most commonly taught and also most commonly represented on board examinations. Other versions involve the physician standing on the same side of the lesion and placing their thenar eminence on the opposite side of the lesion and are segment below.

Strain and Counterstrain for the Thoracic Region

(See Chapter 6 for more detail.)

Key Points

⬚ **Anterior points**—treat with **flexion** and sidebending **toward** lesion.
⬚ **Posterior points**—treat with **extension** and sidebending **away** from lesion.
  ⬚ Anterior—three groups divided by treatment position:
    ⬚ AT1 to AT6 (anterior tenderpoints 1-6)—midline on the sternum. Treat with flexion and arms internally rotated.
    ⬚ AT7 to AT9—abdominal wall, 1 to 2 in lateral to midline between xyphoid and umbilicus. Treat with flexion, sidebending toward, and rotation away from lesion.
    ⬚ AT10 to AT11—abdominal wall below umbilicus. AT12—inner surface of iliac crest at mid-axillary line. Treat with flexion, sidebending, and minimal rotation toward lesion.
  ⬚ Posterior—points can be found on the spinous process (usually the sides) or on the transverse process.
    ⬚ PT1 to PT9 (posterior tenderpoints 1-9)—spinous process of corresponding vertebra. Treat with extension, sidebending, and rotation away from lesion.
    ⬚ PT10 to PT12—spinous process of corresponding vertebra. Treat with extension and rotation toward lesion.
    ⬚ LPT1 to LP12—(lateral posterior tenderpoint)—transverse process of corresponding vertebra. Treat primarily with sidebending away from lesion.

207

ME for Exhaled Ribs 1 or 2 on the Left

(See Figure 9-3.)

- Patient supine, head rotated to the right approximately 30°, with left wrist over forehead. Physician opposite dysfunctional ribs. Top hand is placed over patient's wrist (over the forehead). Bottom hand is placed under angle of dysfunctional rib and continuously exerts an inferior and lateral force.
- Patient is instructed to lift head toward ceiling while the physician resists.
- This is held for 3 to 5 seconds.
- Tissues are then allowed to relax for several seconds, a new barrier engaged, and the process is repeated three to five times.

Muscle energy (ME) uses respiratory assistance—directly pushing the ribs into exhalation—for inhaled ribs. Ribs can also be balanced indirectly to release myofascial restrictions. Elevated first ribs and posterior ribs can be "put back in place" with high velocity, low amplitude (HVLA) and ME techniques. Alternatively, they can be balanced by any of the indirect techniques.

Facilitated Positional Release for Elevated First Rib on the Left

(See Figure 9-4.)

- Patient supine. Physician on side of dysfunction.
- Physician's left hand monitors the patient's rib at its area of greatest tension over the posterior, superior aspect. Physician's right hand manipulates patient's ipsilateral elbow.
- Physician places patient's arm into flexion and internal rotation until tissues around the rib are maximally softened.
- Compression is then added through the elbow in the direction of the monitoring fingers.

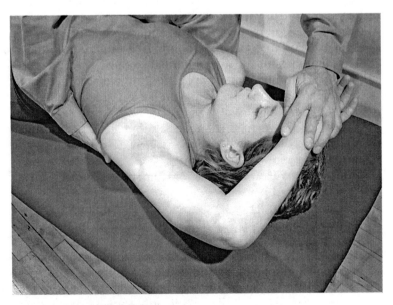

FIGURE 9-3. ME of exhaled ribs 1-2.

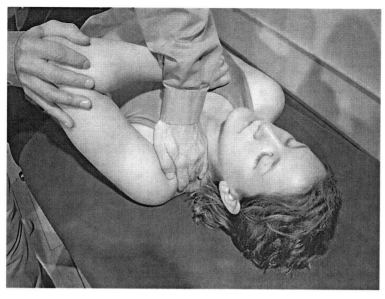

FIGURE 9-4. Facilitated positional release for an elevated first rib.

- Position is held for 3 to 5 seconds.
- While maintaining the current forces, the arm is adducted across the chest and then brought inferiorly and back into neutral in a continuous arc.

In addition, all ribs can be assessed for myofascial restrictions and direct and indirect myofascial release (MFR) techniques used to reduce strain patterns.

Rib Raising

(See Figures 9-5 A and B.)

- Patient lies supine.
- Physician stands to the side of the patient.

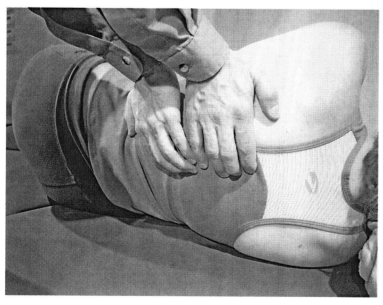

FIGURE 9-5(A). Rib raising.

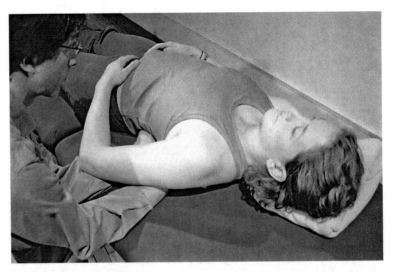

FIGURE 9-5(B). **Rib raising.**

- Physician slides their hands, palms up, so the finger pads contact the rib angles (posterior aspect of the ribs).
- The physician flexes their fingers holding them firmly in place. By using the physician's arms and body as a unit, an upward springing force is applied to the rib cage to exaggerate the patient's inhalation. This is accomplished by the physician locking their fingers, wrists, arms, and shoulders in place with their elbows extended. The physician bends their knees lowering their trunk causing their hands to move upward, articulating the patient's rib cage.
- As the patient exhales, the physician stands up to exaggerate exhalation.
- This cycle is repeated, until motion in the rib cage is improved.
- Reassess, and repeat on opposite side.

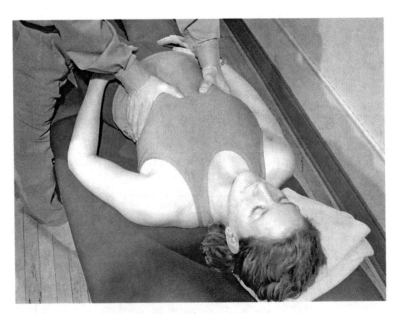

FIGURE 9-6(A). **Indirect balancing of the diaphragm.**

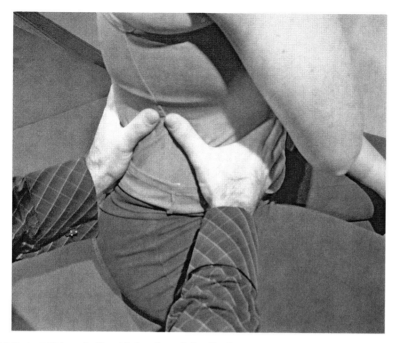

FIGURE 9-6(B).   **Indirect balancing of the diaphragm.**

Indirect Balancing of the Diaphragm

(See Figures 9-6 A and B.)

- The patient is seated or in supine position.
- Physician stands to the side of the patient.
- The physician places one hand under the lower ribs with their fingers between the spinous process of the upper lumbar vertebra. The other hand is placed with the middle finger on the xiphoid process. The rest of the fingers lie inferiorly.
- As the patient breathes, the physician assesses the motion of the hemidiaphragm.
- The physician moves their hands as to follow the direction of least tension of the diaphragm exaggerating this position.
- This position is held through three breathing cycles. After each exhalation, the physician readjusts their hands into the direction of least tension. After three cycles, reassess.
- Repeat this process on the opposite hemidiaphragm.

CHAPTER 10

Lumbar Techniques

High Velocity, Low Amplitude Lateral Recumbent (Posterior Transverse Process Down-Lumbar Low) for a Type II, Flexed Dysfunction, T10 to L5

(See Figure 10-1.)

- Patient is positioned in the **lateral recumbent position** with the side of the dysfunction down (lumbar low).
- Physician stands facing the patient.
- Patient's legs are flexed until motion is palpated at the joint space of the dysfunction.
- Inferior leg is straightened.
- Patient's inferior arm is pulled cephalad and upward to increase rotation of the dysfunctional segment. Patient is asked to look up to the ceiling.
- Physician places caudad forearm over the patient's ilium.
- Physician's cephalad hand monitors the dysfunctional segment.
- Ask patient to inhale/exhale. Physician monitors motion at the dysfunction, while taking up tissue slack. Physician may take up tissue slack with caudad forearm moving the patient's ilium toward the patient's head and downward.
- A high velocity, low amplitude thrust is directed through the physician's caudad forearm toward the patient's head and downward to encourage sidebending.
- Physician's cephalad forearm stabilizes patient's upper torso during the thrust.

For an extended dysfunction, follow the procedure as outlined above. If flexion of the lumbar spine is desired, this can be accomplished by pulling the patient's shoulders anteriorly and not asking the patient to look up.

When performed with the posterior transverse process down, this technique addresses the sidebending component of the dysfunction. For example, if L1 is flexed, rotated, and sidebent to the right, placing the patient on the right side with the patient's left ankle tucked behind their right knee causes left sidebending of the lumbar spine. The final corrective force is an increase in this left sidebending (along with rotation) of the lumbar spine. This technique can be performed with the posterior component up; however, this only addresses the rotational component of the dysfunction.

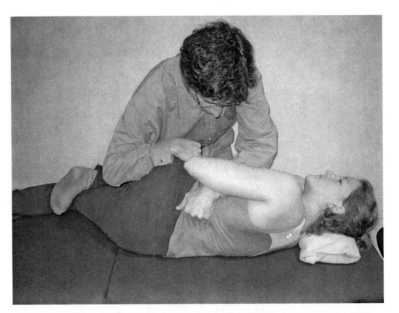

FIGURE 10-1. High velocity, low amplitude lateral recumbent (posterior transverse process down-lumbar low) for a type II, flexed dysfunction, T10-L5.

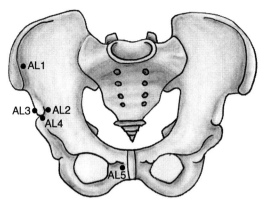

FIGURE 10-2. Anterior lumbar counterstrain tenderpoints.

Counterstrain, Anterior L1 to L5 (AL1-AL5)

TENDERPOINT LOCATION

(See Figure 10-2.)

- **AL1**: Medial side of anterior superior iliac spine (ASIS), press laterally
- **AL2**: Medial side of anterior inferior iliac spine (AIIS), press laterally
- **AL3**: Lateral side of AIIS, press medially
- **AL4**: Inferior side of AIIS, press cephalad
- **AL5**: Anterior surface of pubic rami approximately 1 cm lateral to pubic symphysis and inferior to tubercle, press posteriorly

TREATMENT POSITION

(See Figure 10-3.)

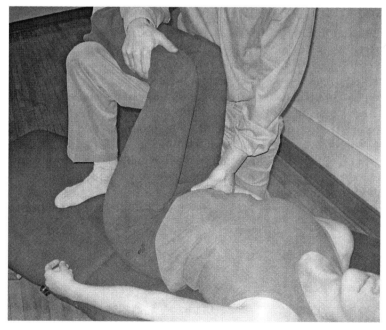

FIGURE 10-3. Counterstrain, anterior L1-L5 (AL1-AL5).

AL1

- Patient is supine.
- Physician stands on same side as the AL1 tenderpoint.
- Tenderpoint is palpated with physician's cephalad hand.
- Physician places caudad leg on table to serve as support for patient's legs.
- Patient's hips are markedly flexed to the level of the L1 vertebrae.
- Patient's legs are placed by physician on physician's caudad leg.
- Patient's feet are pulled toward the tenderpoint side to sidebend the lumbar spine.
- Patient's knees are rotated toward the tenderpoint side to introduce rotation of the L1 segment away form the tenderpoint side.
- Physician monitors the tenderpoint for a maximum decrease in tissue tension and a maximum decrease in tenderness as perceived by the patient.
- Position is held for 90 seconds.
- Physician returns patient's legs to the table without assistance from patient.

AL2 TO AL4

- Patient is supine.
- Physician stands on same side of tenderpoint.
- Physician places caudad leg on table to serve as support for patient's legs.
- Patient's hips are moderately flexed to the level of the dysfunctional vertebrae.
- Patient's legs are placed by physician on physician's caudad leg.
- Patient's knees are rotated toward the tenderpoint, with the amount varying at different vertebral levels.
- Patient is sidebent by moving feet toward from tenderpoint side.
- Physician monitors the tenderpoint for a maximum decrease in tissue tension and a maximum decrease in tenderness as perceived by the patient.
- Position is held for 90 seconds.
- Physician returns patient's legs to the table without assistance from patient.

AL5

- Patient is supine.
- Physician stands on same side of AL5 tenderpoint.
- Physician places caudad leg on table to serve as support for patient's legs.
- Patient's hips are markedly flexed to the level of L5.
- Patient's legs are placed by physician on physician's caudad leg.
- Patient's knees are pulled toward the tenderpoint and patient's feet are moved away from the tenderpoint. This produces sidebending away and torso rotation away from the tenderpoint.
- Physician monitors the tenderpoint for a maximum decrease in tissue tension and a maximum decrease in tenderness as perceived by the patient.
- Position is held for 90 seconds.
- Physician returns patient's legs to the table without assistance from patient.

Counterstrain, Posterior L1 to L5 (PL1-PL5)

TENDERPOINT LOCATION

- **PL1 to PL5:** Inferolateral side of the deviated spinous process which signifies vertebral rotation of this segment to the opposite side

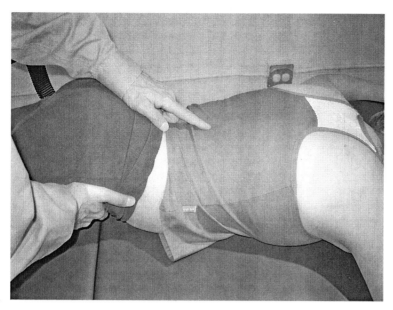

FIGURE 10-4. Counterstrain, posterior L1-L5 (PL1-PL5).

TREATMENT POSITION

(See Figure 10-4.)

PL1 TO PL5

- Patient is **prone**.
- Physician stands on the same side of posterior tenderpoint.
- Physician extends patient's trunk on the same side of the tender by lifting the pelvis posteriorly, which creates extension and rotation of the lower vertebrae toward the tenderpoint side.
- Physician monitors the tenderpoint for a maximum decrease in tissue tension and a maximum decrease in tenderness as perceived by the patient.
- Position is held for 90 seconds.
- Physician returns patient to neutral position without assistance from patient.

Facilitated Positional Release, Extended Somatic Dysfunction

(See Figure 10-5.)

- Patient is prone with the side of the somatic dysfunction close to the edge of the table.
- Place pillows under the abdomen to cause flattening of the lumbar lordosis.
- Physician stands facing the head of the table on the same side of the patient's dysfunction.
- A pillow is placed under the patient's thigh on the side of the dysfunction.
- Physician monitors the posterior transverse process of the dysfunctional lumbar vertebrae with the hand closest to the patient.
- Physician uses the other hand to abduct patient's leg on the same side as the dysfunction creating lumbar sidebending (physician stands between table and patient's abducted leg).

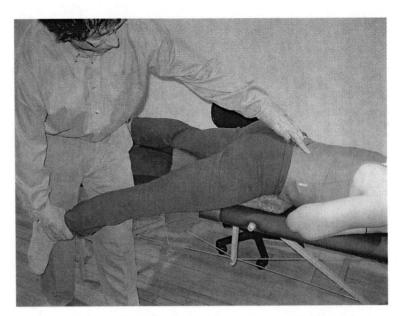

FIGURE 10-5. Facilitated positional release, extended somatic dysfunction.

- Physician internally rotates patient's abducted leg until motion is palpated under physician's monitoring finger.
- Physician flexes patient's hip by moving the abducted leg toward the floor.
- With the pillow acting as a fulcrum, the physician lifts the patient's pelvis from the table introducing lumbar extension.
- Physician holds this position until a release is appreciated, usually 3 to 5 seconds.
- Physician slowly returns the patient to neutral without assistance from the patient.

Facilitated Positional Release, Flexed Somatic Dysfunction

(See Figure 10-6.)

- Patient is prone with the side of the somatic dysfunction close to the edge of the table.
- Place pillows under the abdomen to cause flattening of the lumbar lordosis.
- Physician sits facing the head of the table on the same side of the patient's dysfunction.
- Physician monitors the posterior transverse process of the dysfunctional lumbar vertebrae with the hand closest to the patient.
- Physician flexes patient's leg (on the side of the dysfunction) at the knee and the hip, resting the lower leg between their legs, creating flexion of the spine until motion is palpated at the site of the dysfunction.
- The physician then abducts the knee until motion is appreciated at the somatic dysfunction.
- The physician holds and supports the knee throughout the remainder of the technique.
- Physician then rotates their body clockwise to introduce rotation.
- Compression can be added through the patient's knee.
- Physician holds this position until a release is appreciated, usually 3 to 5 seconds.
- Physician slowly returns the patient to neutral without assistance from the patient.

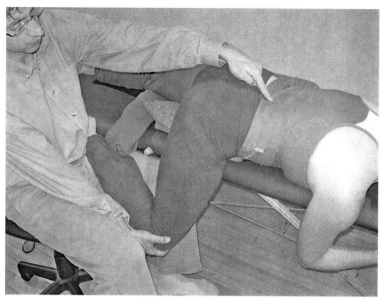

FIGURE 10-6. Facilitated positional release, flexed somatic dysfunction.

High Velocity, Low Amplitude: Leg Pull Dysfunction: Short Leg

(See Figure 10-7.)

- With the patient lying supine and the physician standing at the foot of the bed, the physician holds onto the patient's ankle. The patient is asked to hold onto the sides of the table.
- Next, the physician gently leans backward applying a traction force onto the patient's leg.
- The physician then slowly abducts the leg until a restrictive barrier is met.
- Slight internal rotation is then applied to the leg by rotating the ankle medially, so to gap the sacroiliac (SI) joint.
- The corrective force is applied as the physician forcefully tugs on the patient's leg.
- Reassess.

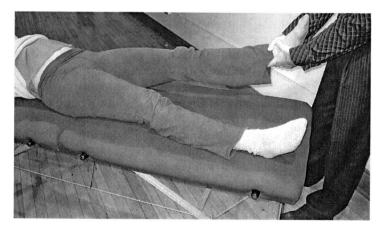

FIGURE 10-7. High velocity, low amplitude: leg pull dysfunction: short leg.

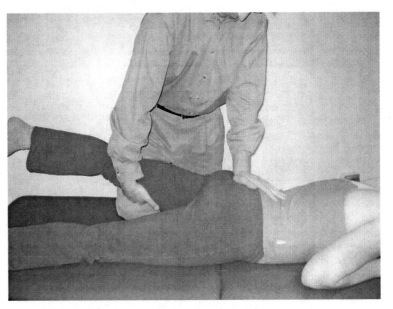

FIGURE 10-8. Muscle energy—psoas muscle spasm.

Muscle Energy—Psoas Muscle Spasm

(See Figure 10-8.)

- The patient lies prone.
- The physician stands at the side of the table on the side of the tight psoas.
- The physician stabilizes the patient's lumbar paravertebral area with their cephalad hand.
- With their caudad hand, the physician grasps the patient's leg, proximal to the knee, and extends the leg at the hip.
- The physician asks the patient to gently push their knee down toward the table for 3 to 5 seconds and then to relax.
- The physician reengages the barrier and repeats the above sequence.
- Reassess.

Muscle Energy—Lumbar Walk Around for a Type II, Flexed Dysfunction, L1 to L5

- Patient is positioned straddling the table with their back at the edge of the table.
- Physician stands at the end of the table facing the patient's back.
- Patient is instructed to cross their arms over the chest and slump forward.
- Physician places their thenar eminence of the hand on the side of the posterior component directly on the posterior component with the physician's elbow locked into their own flank to provide support. The physician's opposite arm is placed across the chest of the patient with the physician's axilla superior to the patient shoulder and the physician's hand on the opposite shoulder, ipsilateral to the posterior component.
- Physician applies an anterior force (toward the patient's umbilicus) to the posterior component to move the dysfunctional segment into extension. This extension is maintained throughout the technique.

LUMBAR TECHNIQUES

OSTEOPATHIC TREATMENTS AND TECHNIQUES

- Physician introduces sidebending to the dysfunctional segment by translating the segment into the restrictive barrier and applying a downward force through the patient's shoulder from the physician's axilla. This sidebending is maintained throughout the technique.
- Next, the physician introduces rotation to the dysfunctional segment by rotating the segment around into the restrictive barrier. This is accomplished by applying rotation through the physician's thenar eminence to the posterior component and shuffling their feet to walk the segment around into the barrier. **Important:** The physician must maintain the extension and sidebending component while adding rotation.
- Once the restrictive barrier is engaged for all three planes of motion, the patient is asked to sidebend and rotate away from the barrier. This is accomplished by asking the patient to lift up their shoulder into the physician's axilla and to rotate into the physician's thenar eminence for 3 to 5 seconds, while the physician resists these two motions. The patient then is asked to relax.
- The physician waits 1 to 2 seconds and then reengages the barrier and repeats the above sequence until motion within the segment is improved.
- The physician should then reassess.

CHAPTER 11

Sacrum and Pelvis Techniques

Muscle Energy for Forward Torsion

(See Figure 11-1.)

- Patient is positioned on side of involved axis (left side for left on left forward torsion).
- Physician stands facing the patient.
- Patient is asked to "hug" the table.
- Patient's superior shoulder is brought as close to the table as possible.
- Patient's hips and knees are flexed 90° or until there is gapping at the lumbosacral junction. This is monitored by the physician's cephalad hand.

PART 1

- Patient is positioned on the side of involved axis (left side for left on left forward torsion). The physician places caudad hand to hold the patient's knees and hips in position and places cephalad hand over the patient's scapula which is closest to the physician.
- As the patient is "hugging" the table, the patient is asked to inhale and during exhalation reach to the floor with their arm which is closest to the physician. During this exhalation phase, the physician follows this motion with their cephalad hand pushing the patient's shoulder toward the floor through scapular pressure.
- Patient then repeats the cycle of inhalation and exhalation three to five times or until no further improvement in rotation of L5 is demonstrated. During inhalation the physician maintains constant pressure over the scapula.

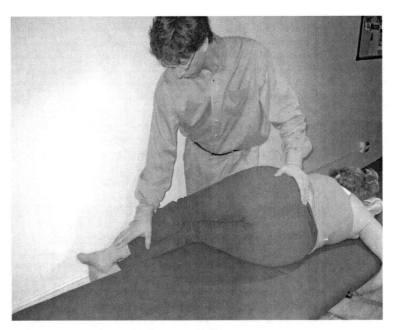

FIGURE 11-1. **Muscle energy for forward torsion.**

Part 2

- Patient is positioned on side of involved axis (left side for left on left forward torsion). The physician places caudad hand to hold the patient's knees and hips in position and places cephalad hand at the patient's lumbosacral junction to monitor.
- Patient's legs are brought off the table.
- Physician places hand on upper leg just proximal to lateral malleolus.
- Patient is instructed to raise legs toward ceiling.
- Physician counters patient's force for 3 to 5 seconds.
- Patient is told to relax; physician waits 1 to 2 seconds.
- Patient's legs are brought further toward the floor.
- The final four steps are repeated three to five times or until no further improvement is demonstrated in sidebending of the sacrum.

Muscle Energy Technique for Backward Torsion

(See Figure 11-2.)

- Patient is positioned on side of involved axis (left side for right on left backward torsion).
- Physician stands facing the patient.
- Patient's superior shoulder is brought posteriorly until restrictive barrier is reached.
- Patient's hips are flexed to 45° while knees are flexed to 90° or until there is gapping at the lumbosacral junction.
- Patient's upper leg is brought off the table while lower leg remains on the table.
- Physician places hand on upper leg of the patient just proximal to lateral malleolus.
- Patient is instructed to raise upper leg toward ceiling.

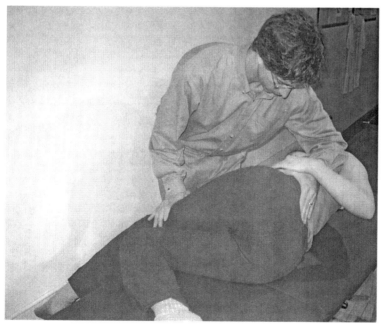

FIGURE 11-2. Muscle energy technique for backward torsion.

- Physician counters patient's force for 3 to 5 seconds.
- Patient is told to relax; physician waits 1 to 2 seconds.
- Patient's upper leg is brought further toward the floor.
- The final four steps are repeated three to five times or until no further improvement is demonstrated in sidebending of the sacrum.

High Velocity, Low Amplitude Technique for Anterior Sacrum

(See Figure 11-3.)

- Patient is positioned on opposite side of dysfunction (left side for a right anterior sacrum) such that the dysfunctional sacroiliac (SI) joint is up (sacrum supreme).
- Patient's hips and knees are flexed until motion is detected at dysfunctional SI joint.
- Patient's upper leg is brought off the table.
- Physician's cephalad hand monitors the dysfunctional SI joint while the cephalad forearm places posterior force on patient's upper shoulder to stabilize the patient.
- Physician's caudad forearm is placed over the ilium just anterior to the dysfunctional SI joint.
- A quick, gentle thrust is applied to the patient's ilium rotating the ilium in an anterior position from behind.

High Velocity, Low Amplitude Technique for Posterior Sacrum

(See Figure 11-4.)

- Patient is positioned supine.
- Physician stands on opposite side of dysfunction (left side for a right posterior sacrum) facing patient.
- Patient either crosses their arms on their chest or interlaces fingers behind their neck.

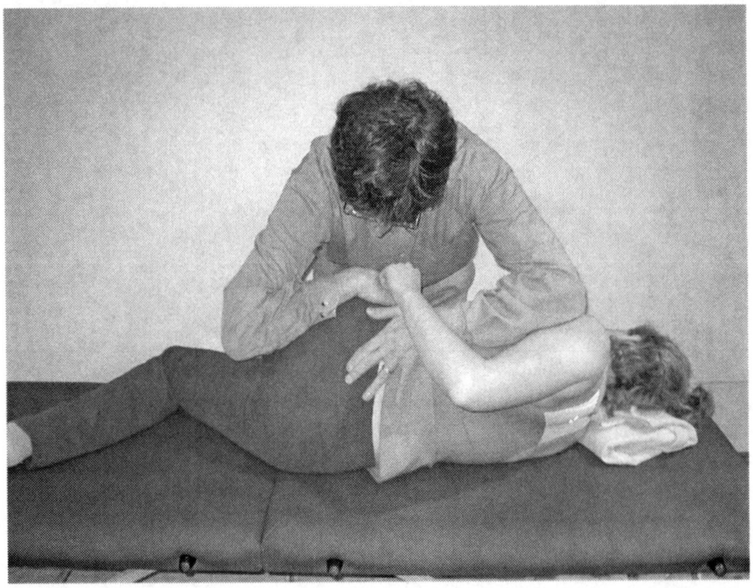

FIGURE 11-3. High velocity, low amplitude technique for anterior sacrum.

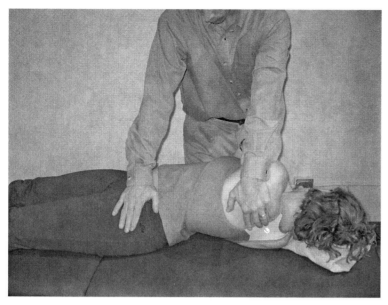

FIGURE 11-4. High velocity, low amplitude technique for posterior sacrum.

- Physician moves patient's shoulders such that the torso is sidebent to the side of the dysfunctional SI joint (making a smiley face with the patient's torso) and places the patient's shoulders perpendicular to the table so the shoulders are rotated away from the dysfunctional SI joint.
- Physician places caudad hand on the opposite anterior superior iliac spine (ASIS) and rotates it downward/away until the restrictive barrier is achieved. The physician's cephalad hand stabilizes the upper torso. There is no rotation applied to the upper torso.
- A quick, gentle thrust is applied to the patient's ilium on the side of the dysfunctional SI joint with the physician's caudad hand on the ASIS. The physician's cephalad hand maintains the position of the patient's upper torso.

Muscle Energy Technique for Anterior Innominate

(See Figure 11-5.)

- Patient is positioned supine.
- Patient's knee and hip are flexed such that knee is brought to patient's chest on side of anterior ilium.
- Physician contacts patient's knee while stabilizing patient's pelvis. If necessary, physician contacts both sides of the table, while patient's knee is brought into physician's axilla.
- Patient is instructed to push knee into physician's hand/axilla, while physician maintains counterforce for 3 to 5 seconds.
- Patient is told to relax.
- Physician waits 1 to 2 seconds and then engages the new restrictive barrier.
- Final three steps are repeated three to five times or until further improvement is demonstrated.

Muscle Energy Technique for Posterior Innominate

(See Figure 11-6.)

- Patient is positioned prone.
- Physician stands on opposite side of dysfunction.

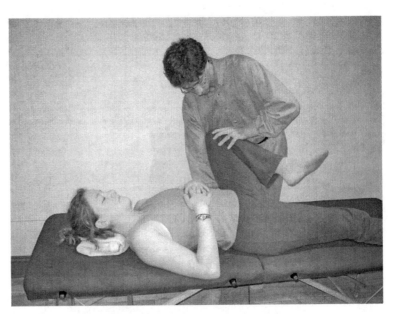

FIGURE 11-5. Muscle energy technique for anterior innominate.

- Patient's knee is flexed 90°.
- Physician contacts patient's thigh just proximal to the knee.
- Patient's hip is passively extended while patient's SI joint is stabilized.
- Patient is asked to push knee into physician's hand while physician maintains counterforce for 3 to 5 seconds.
- Patient is told to relax.
- Physician waits 1 to 2 seconds and then engages the new restrictive barrier.
- Final three steps are repeated three to five times or until further improvement is demonstrated.

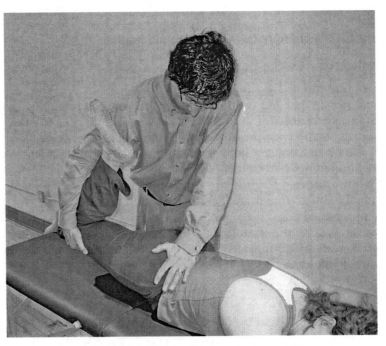

FIGURE 11-6. Muscle energy technique for posterior innominate.

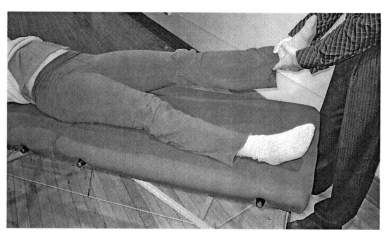

FIGURE 11-7. High velocity, low amplitude technique for innominate up-slip.

High Velocity, Low Amplitude Technique for Innominate Up-Slip

(See Figure 11-7.)

- Patient is positioned supine.
- Physician stands at patient's feet.
- Physician holds ankle on the side of dysfunction.
- Physician applies a traction force to the leg from the ankle to the hip.
- Physician slightly flexes and internally rotates leg.
- A quick, gentle thrust is applied to leg by increasing traction from ankle.

Extremity Techniques

Muscle Energy for Shoulder

(See Figure 12-1.)

- Patient sits on table with physician standing behind.
- Range of motion is tested in all directions.
- Decreased range of motion is noted.
- The restrictive barrier is engaged.
- The patient performs three to five repetitions of 3 to 5 seconds isometric contraction against the physician's resistance.
- The range of motion is reassessed for improvement.

Articulatory—Spencer Seven-Step Technique

- Patient lies in the lateral recumbent position with affected shoulder up.
- The physician stands behind or facing the patient.
- The physician stabilizes the clavicle and scapula (shoulder girdle).
    - **Step one:** The physician gently extends the arm in the sagittal plane with the elbow flexed. Repetitions are made according to the patient's comfort level (see Figure 12-2 A).
    - **Step two:** The physician flexes the patient's arm in the sagittal plane, with the elbow extended, and induces a rhythmic, swinging movement, increasing range so that the patient's arm covers the ear (see Figure 12-2 B).
    - **Step three:** The physician circumducts the patient's abducted humerus with the elbow flexed. The physician makes clockwise and counterclockwise concentric circles, gradually increasing the range within limits of pain (see Figure 12-2 C).
    - **Step four:** The physician circumducts the patient's humerus with the elbow extended. The physician makes clockwise and counterclockwise circles with the arm, increasing range as permitted by the patient's pain tolerance (see Figure 12-2 D).

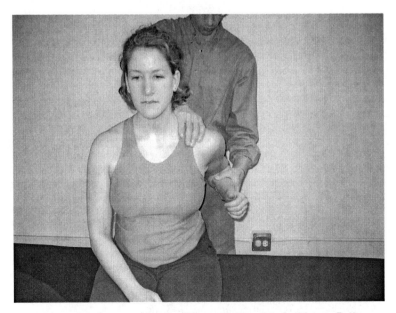

FIGURE 12-1. Muscle energy for shoulder, patient resisted with arm flexion.

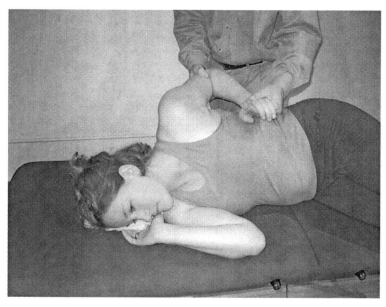

FIGURE 12-2(A). Spencer technique—step 1, arm extension.

- **Step five:** The physician abducts the patient's arm with the elbow flexed and gradually increases the range of abduction against the stabilized shoulder girdle (see Figure 12-2 E).
- **Step six:** The physician places the patient's hand behind the rib cage and gently springs the elbow forward and inferior, increasing internal rotation of the humerus (see Figure 12-2 F).
- **Step seven:** The physician grasps the patient's proximal humerus with both hands and applies a lateral and caudad traction in a pumping fashion (see Figure 12-2 G).
- Retest.

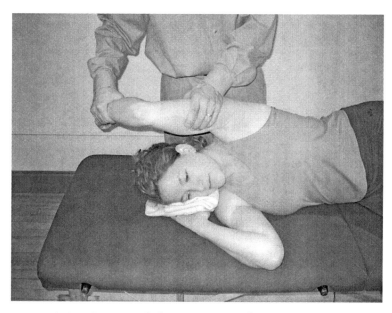

FIGURE 12-2(B). Spencer technique—step 2, arm flexion.

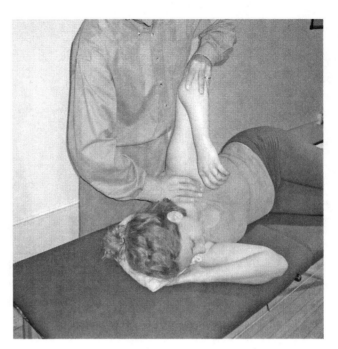

FIGURE 12-2(C). Spencer technique—step 3, circumduction with elbow flexion.

Counterstrain—Coracoid Tenderpoint Counterstrain Technique

(See Figure 12-3.)

- The physician stands behind the seated patient.
- The physician finds a tenderpoint located over the coracoid process, at the insertion of pectoralis minor and the short head of the biceps, with the cephalad hand.

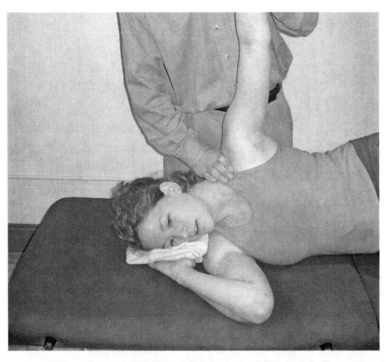

FIGURE 12-2(D). Spencer technique—step 4, circumduction with elbow extension.

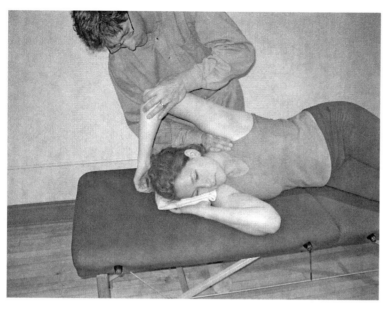

FIGURE 12-2(E). Spencer technique—step 5, arm abduction.

- The physician flexes the patient's arm at the elbow with the caudad hand, unloading the biceps and loading the triceps.
- The physician protracts the shoulder to shorten pectoralis minor.
- The physician monitors the tenderpoint for 90 seconds, palpating for a release.

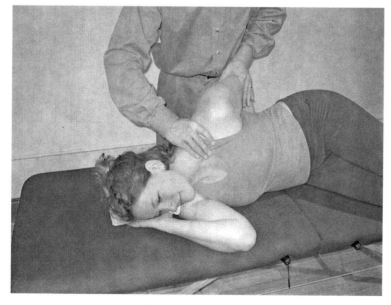

FIGURE 12-2(F). Spencer technique—step 6, arm internal rotation.

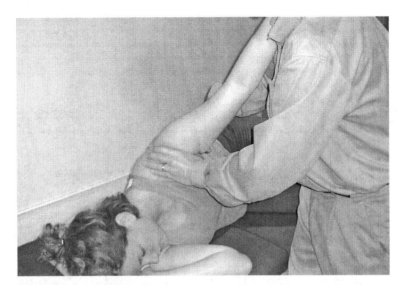

FIGURE 12-2(G). Spencer technique—step 7, arm traction.

High Velocity, Low Amplitude—Thrust Technique for Anterior Radial Head and Posterior Radial Head

(See Figures 12-4, 12-5.)

- The physician stands facing the seated patient.
- For anterior radial head dysfunction, the physician grasps the dysfunctional arm and flexes the arm at the elbow while adding pronation at the wrist.
- The physician places the second and third digits of his other hand into the crease of the patient's elbow, directly over the radial head.
- The physician exerts a rapid hyperflexion force on the elbow while simultaneously thrusting the radial head dorsally with the fingers of the other hand.

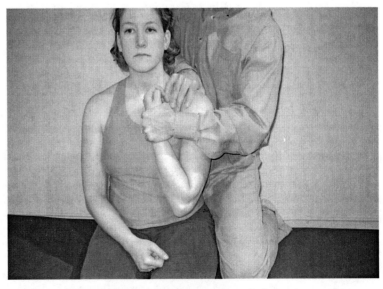

FIGURE 12-3. Coracoid tenderspot counterstrain technique.

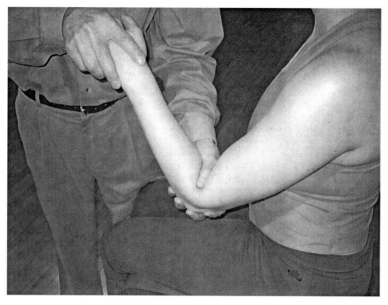

FIGURE 12-4. Technique for anterior radial head dysfunction.

- For a posterior radial head dysfunction, the physician grasps the patient's arm at the elbow and extends it.
- The physician places their thumbs over the head of the radius posteriorly and the phalanx of the index finger over the radial head anteriorly.
- The physician exerts a rapid hyperextension force on the patient's elbow, while simultaneously inducing a ventral counterforce through the radial head.

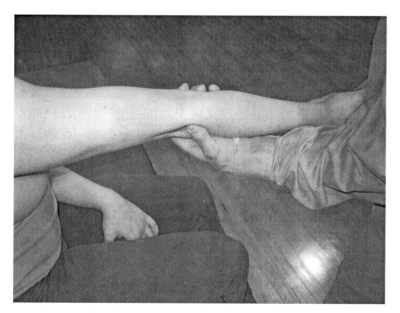

FIGURE 12-5. Technique for posterior radial head dysfunction.

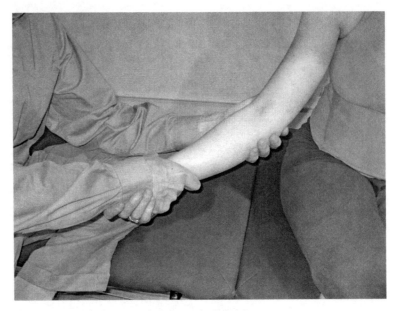

FIGURE 12-6. Technique for restriction in supination.

Muscle Energy—Supination and Pronation Dysfunction

(See Figure 12-6.)

- The physician stands in front of the seated patient.
- The physician flexes the patient's elbow to 90° and stabilizes the joint with his medial hand. The lateral hand grasps the distal forearm, wrist, and hand with the thumb pointed vertically.
- The physician induces supination and pronation, testing for dysfunction and comparing to the opposite side.
- To treat supination dysfunction, the physician stabilizes the elbow and monitors the radial head with the lateral hand, while the medial hand supinates the forearm to the resistant barrier.
- The patient performs three to five contractions for 3 to 5 seconds against resistance offered by the physician's medial hand.
- The physician engages a new supination barrier after each patient contraction.
- Treatment of pronation dysfunction involves the same hand placement, but engages the barrier in pronation.
- The patient performs three to five contractions for 3 to 5 seconds against resistance offered by the physician's medial hand.
- The physician engages a new pronation barrier after each patient contraction.
- The physician reassesses.

Counterstrain—Lateral Epicondyle Tenderpoints

(See Figure 12-7.)

- The patient is seated.
- The physician stands on the side of affected extremity.
- The physician palpates the tenderpoint over the lateral epicondyle.
- With his other hand, the physician flexes the elbow and places the wrist in extension. The physician fine-tunes the position with supination or pronation.

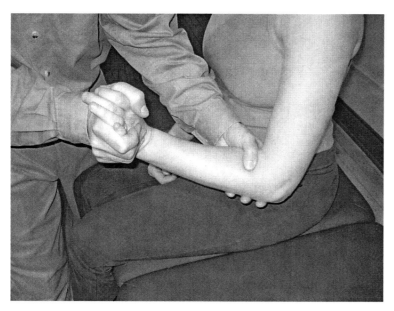

FIGURE 12-7. Counterstrain for lateral epicondyle tenderpoint.

* The position is held for 90 seconds.
* The arm is slowly returned to a neutral position.

Muscle Energy—Wrist Restriction in Radial Deviation

(See Figure 12-8.)

* The joint is moved into the barrier of radial deviation.
* The patient is asked to push toward the ulnar aspect against physician resistance. The contraction is held for 3 to 5 seconds.

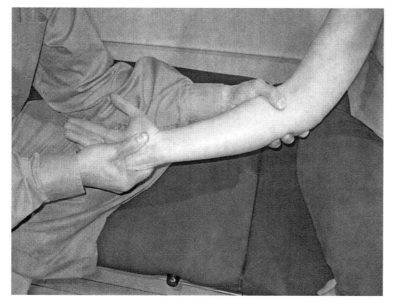

FIGURE 12-8. Muscle energy for wrist restriction in radial deviation.

- The joint is moved into a new barrier.
- The technique is repeated three more times.

Counterstrain—To Treat Wrist Tenderpoints

(See Figure 12-9.)

- The physician finds the tenderpoint on the dorsal or ventral aspect of the wrist. The physician flexes or extends the wrist around the tenderpoint.
- The physician holds the position for 90 seconds.
- The physician returns the wrist to neutral and reassesses the tenderpoint.

Articulatory Treatment for the Hand

(See Figure 12-10.)

- The physician locks one metacarpal between the thumb and index finger of one hand.
- With the thumb and index finger of the other hand, the physician moves the adjacent metacarpal into rotation and anterior or posterior glide.

Counterstrain—Piriformis

(See Figure 12-11.)

- The patient lies prone and the physician stands on the side of the tight piriformis. The patient locates the piriformis tenderpoint with his cephalad hand.
- The physician grasps the patient's leg with their caudad hand and flexes the patient's knee to 90°.
- The physician abducts the leg and externally rotates the leg.

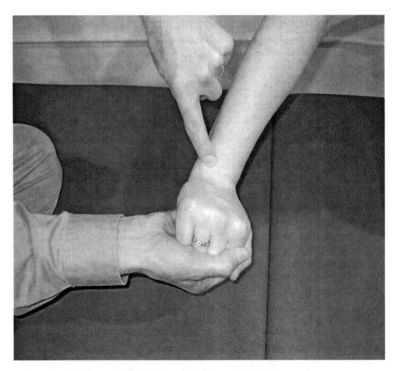

FIGURE 12-9. Counterstrain for dorsal wrist tenderpoint.

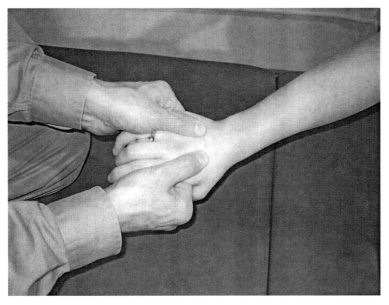

FIGURE 12-10. **Metacarpal articulation.**

- The physician reassesses the tenderpoint.
- The physician holds the position for 90 seconds and slowly returns the leg to neutral.
- The physician reassesses the tenderpoint.

High Velocity, Low Amplitude—Anterior Fibular Head Dysfunction

(See Figure 12-12.)

- The patient lies supine.
- The physician stands by the table on the same side as the dysfunction.
- The physician grasps the patient's foot on the side of the somatic dysfunction with the nonthrusting hand.
- The physician places the thenar eminence of their thrusting hand on the anterior superior aspect of the fibular head.

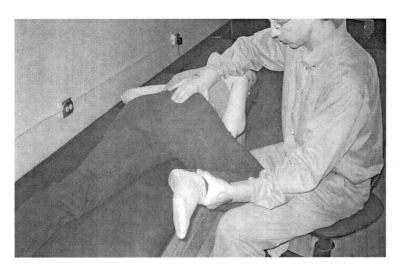

FIGURE 12-11. **Piriformis counterstrain technique.**

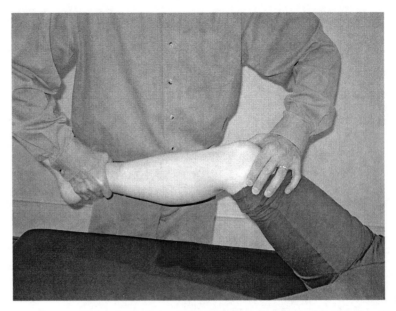

FIGURE 12-12. High velocity, low amplitude for anterior fibular head dysfunction.

* The patient's knee is gently flexed.
* The physician extends the patient's knee rapidly, while simultaneously introducing a downward and medial thrust through the fibular head.

Counterstrain—Patellar Tenderpoint

(See Figure 12-13.)

* The patient lies supine.
* The physician stands beside the table.
* A rolled pillow is placed below the patient's calf.

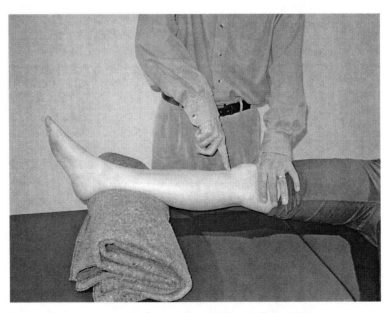

FIGURE 12-13. Counterstrain for anterior patellar tenderpoint.

- The knee is hyperextended as the physician presses down on the anterior thigh, proximal to the patella.
- The foot is internally rotated.

Counterstrain—Medial Ankle Tenderpoint

(See Figure 12-14.)

- The patient lies on their side with the affected leg up.
- The physician sits beside the table.
- The physician takes the affected foot off the table and a towel is placed under the anterior ankle.
- The physician inverts the foot, pressing forcefully on the lateral side of the foot.
- The physician holds the foot for 90 seconds following traditional counterstrain technique.

High Velocity, Low Amplitude—Cuboid and Navicular Somatic Dysfunction

(See Figure 12-15.)

- The patient lies prone.
- The physician stands beside the table on the side of the dysfunction.
- The physician drops the dysfunctional leg off the side of the table and flexes the patient's hip and knee.
- The physician grasps the patient's foot with both hands and places their thumbs in a "V" shape over the cuboid or navicular.
- The physician exerts a downward thrust through their thumbs while simultaneously inducing a whip-like action at the patient's ankle and knee.

Articulation—Metatarsal Heads

(See Figure 12-16.)

- The patient lies supine.
- The physician stands at the end of the table.

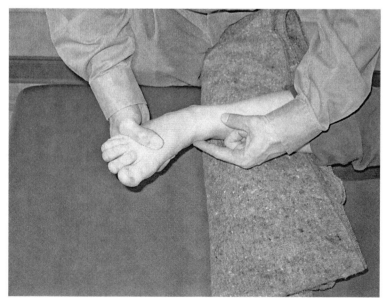

FIGURE 12-14. Medial ankle tenderpoint counterstrain.

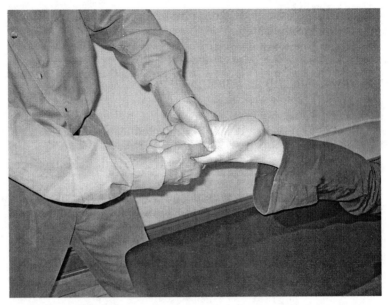

FIGURE 12-15. High velocity, low amplitude for navicular somatic dysfunction, performed with patient prone.

- The physician grasps the shaft of the second metatarsal with the medial hand and the shaft of the third metatarsal with the lateral hand.
- The physician moves the second metatarsal dorsally and ventrally to increase mobility.

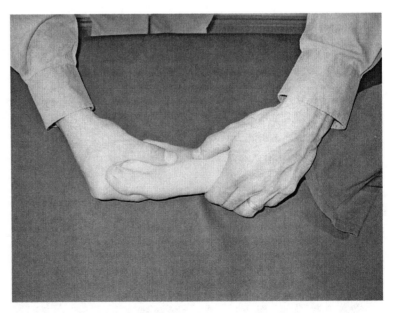

FIGURE 12-16. Metatarsal articulation.

Systemic Techniques

Sinus Technique

INHIBITORY PRESSURE OF THE THREE BRANCHES OF THE TRIGEMINAL NERVE TO IMPROVE DRAINAGE OF THE RESPIRATORY SINUSES

(See Figure 13-1.)

- The physician lies at the head of the table.
- The patient lies supine.
- The physician locates the supraorbital foramen above the orbits bilaterally.
- The physician applies gentle, alternating pressure to the area for approximately 3 to 5 seconds.
- The physician performs the same motion to the infraorbital foramen on the maxilla and the mental foramen on the mandible.

VOMER PUMP

(See Figure 13-2.)

- The physician stands by the side of the table, next to the patient's head.
- The patient lies supine.
- The physician places their gloved index finger of the caudad hand inside the patient's mouth contacting the intermaxillary suture line.
- The physician places the cephalad index finger over the frontonasal articulation.
- The patient gently closes their mouth.
- The physician presses in a cephalad direction in a rhythmic fashion.
- The physician feels for motion at the frontonasal articulation.
- Upon feeling motion, the physician stops the technique.

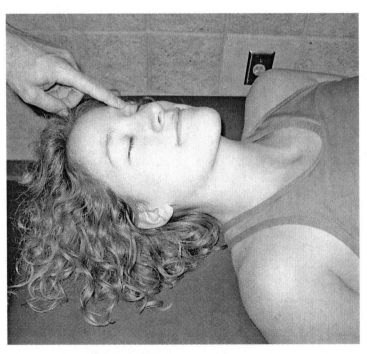

FIGURE 13-1. Sinus technique inhibitory pressure.

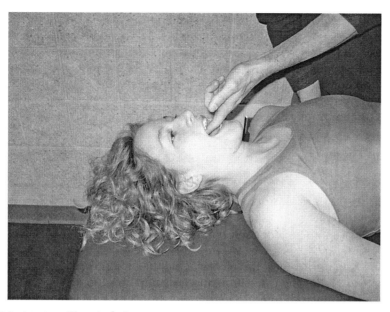

FIGURE 13-2. Sinus technique: vomer pump.

MANDIBULAR DRAINAGE TECHNIQUE FOR OTITIS MEDIA—GALBREATH TECHNIQUE

(See Figure 13-3.)

- The patient is seated or lies supine, her head tilted to 30° and turned with the affected ear up.
- The physician is seated at the side of the table, adjacent to the patient's head, looking directly at the patient.

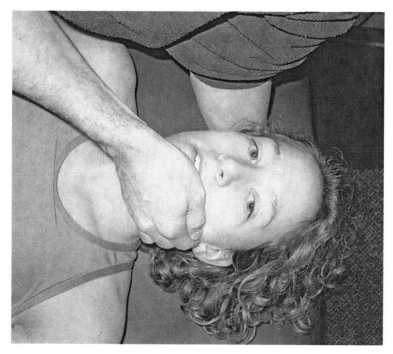

FIGURE 13-3. Mandibular drainage technique for otitis media—Galbreath technique.

- The physician's cephalad hand is placed on the patient's occiput.
- The physician's caudad hand is placed on the patient's mandible with the index and middle finger on the condyle of the mandible.
- The physician applies a gentle pressure with the caudad hand, pushing the condyle down and inward, and drawing the mandible toward the physician. The pressure is released.
- The motion is repeated every 3 to 5 seconds over 30 to 60 seconds.

LYMPHATIC PUMP

(See Figure 13-4.)

- With the patient supine and the physician standing at the head of the patient, the physician places their hand on the patient's thoracic wall, with the thenar eminence of each hand inferior to the respective clavicle. The fingers are spread apart.
- As the patient breathes, the physician applies a compressive force through their arms, following exhalation and resisting inhalation.
- This is continued through 3 to 4 cycles, resisting inhalation and following exhalation.
- One-third of the way through the fourth inhalation, quickly remove your hands from the patient's thoracic wall. This causes a negative intrathoracic pressure within the thoracic cavity, assisting flow.

PEDAL LYMPHATIC PUMP

(See Figure 13-5.)

- The patient lies supine.
- The physician stands at the foot of the table.
- The physician grabs the soles of the patient's feet, and dorsiflexes them.
- The physician applies an oscillatory dorsiflexion force through the longitudinal axis of the patient's body, at a rate of about 2 to 3 forces per second.
- The physician can continue the force for up to 5 to 10 minutes.

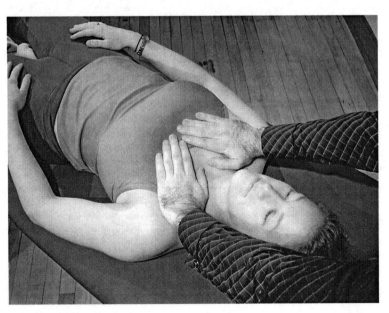

FIGURE 13-4.   Lymphatic pump.

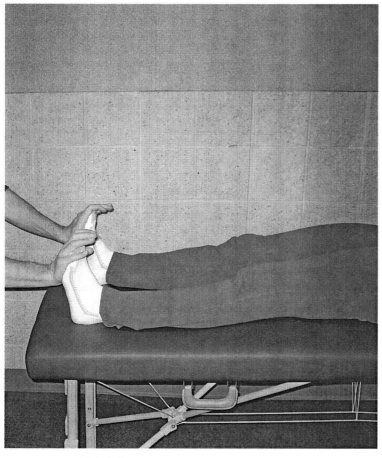

FIGURE 13-5. Pedal lymphatic pump.

MYOFASCIAL RELEASE OF THE THORACIC OUTLET

(See Figure 13-6.)

- With the patient lying supine and the physician seated at the head of the patient, the physician places both hands on either side of the patient's neck. The thumbs are placed posterior to the neck; the thenar eminence is superior to the superior border of the scapula.
- The fingers are spread apart and placed inferior to the clavicle on each side. Contact is light so as to assess motion of the fascia.
- Assess the motion in all planes.
- Once the position of least tension is achieved, hold that position until a release is felt.
- Return to neutral and reassess.

Techniques for the Gastrointestinal Tract

MESENTERIC LIFT (SMALL INTESTINE, CECUM)

(See Figure 13-7.)

- Patient position = supine.
- Patient places feet on table by bending knees to relax abdomen.
- Physician gently "scoops" viscera in area of focus toward mesenteric attachment.
- Tissues are held until a sense of relaxation is palpated.

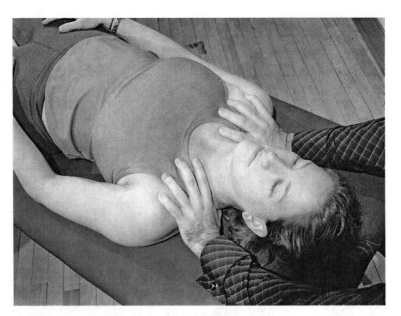

FIGURE 13-6. Myofascial release of the thoracic outlet.

General Lower Abdominal/Pelvic Lift

(See Figure 13-8.)

- Patient position = supine.
- Patient places feet on table by bending knees to relax abdomen.
- Physician places hands over viscera in area of focus, keeping fingers flat.

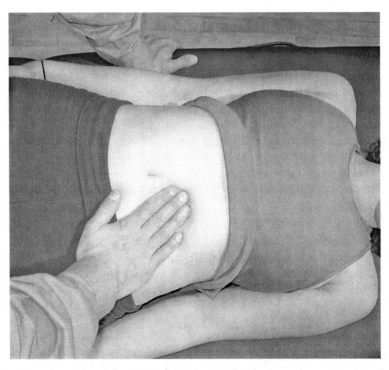

FIGURE 13-7. Mesenteric lift (small intestine, cecum).

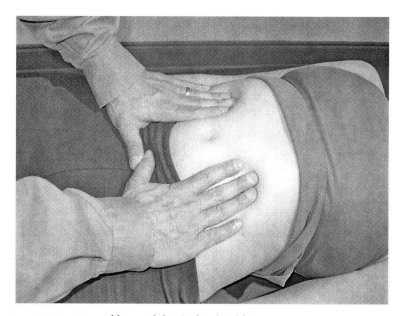

FIGURE 13-8. General lower abdominal/pelvic lift.

- Viscera are lifted superiorly, until an area of restriction is noted.
- Maintain lift until tissues release.

Treatment of Anterior Chapman Reflexes for the Colon

- Patient position = supine.
- Chapman reflexes for the colon are located along the iliotibial band, in relation to the mirror image of the colonic anatomical structures they represent (see Chapman diagram, Figure 6-7)
- Once a Chapman point is localized, firm pressure is applied to the point.
- Pressure is applied in a circular pattern with the attempt to flatten the mass.
- Continue pressure until the mass disappears, or until the patient can no longer tolerate the procedure.

PUBIC SYMPHYSIS COMPRESSION

MUSCLE ENERGY

(See Figure 13-9.)

- With the patient lying supine and the physician standing on the side of the patient so that the dominant hand is caudad, the physician has the patient flex their legs so that the feet are flat on the table.
- The physician places their dominant arm between the patient's medial aspects of their knees, with the elbow contacting the medial aspect of one knee and the thenar eminence contacting the medial aspect of the other knee.
- The physician's opposite hand is placed on the anterior/superior aspect of the patient's pelvis for stabilization.
- The patient is instructed to abduct their knees together against the wedge created by your forearm.

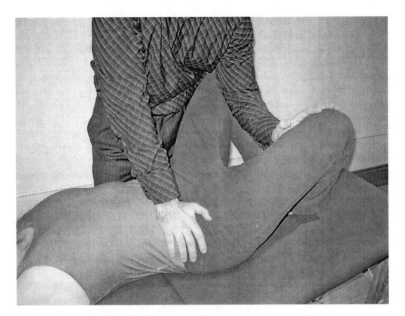

FIGURE 13-9. Pubic symphysis compression.

- This position is held for 3 to 5 seconds.
- The patient relaxes for 3 seconds.
- These steps are repeated three to five times.
- Reassess.

Techniques for the Hospitalized Patient

See rib raising (Chapter 9, Figure 9-5 A and B) and pedal lymphatic pump (earlier in this chapter).

Abbreviations

Abbreviation	Meaning
AIIS	anterior inferior iliac spine
ANS	autonomic nervous system
AOA	American Osteopathic Association
AP	anteroposterior
ART	articulation
ASIS	anterior superior iliac spine
ATFL	anterior talofibular ligament
BPH	benign prostatic hyperplasia
BLT	balanced ligamentous tension
CABG	coronary artery bypass graft
CE	cognitive evaluation
CFL	calcaneofibular ligament
CHF	congestive heart failure
CN	cranial nerve
COMLEX	Comprehensive Osteopathic Medical Licensing Examination
COPD	chronic obstructive pulmonary disease
CRI	cranial rhythmic impulse
CRP	Chapman reflex point(s)
CS	counterstrain
CSF	cerebrospinal fluid
CT	computerized tomography
CV	cardiovascular
DA	deep articulation
DJD	degenerative joint disease
DOE	dyspnea on exertion
ER	emergency room
FHT	fetal heart tones
FPR	facilitated positional release
GI	gastrointestinal
GU	genitourinary
H&P	history and physical
HA	headache
HEENT	head, ears, eyes, nose, throat
HVLA	high velocity, low amplitude
ILA	inferior lateral angle
ITB	iliotibial band
IUP	intrauterine pregnancy

Abbreviation	Meaning
IVC	inferior vena cava
MC	metacarpal
MCP	metacarpophalangeal (joint)
ME	muscle energy
MFR	myofascial release
MI	myocardial infarction
MVA	motor vehicle accident
NBOME	National Board of Osteopathic Medical Examiners
NSVD	normal spontaneous vaginal delivery
OA	occipitoatlantal
OCP	oral contraceptive pills
OMM	osteopathic manipulative medicine
OMT	osteopathic manipulative techniques
PE	performance evaluation
PMS	premenstrual syndrome
PRM	primary respiratory mechanism
PSIS	posterior superior iliac spines
PT	physical therapy
PTFL	posterior talofibular ligament
ROM	range of motion
RTM	reciprocal tension membrane
SBR	sidebending rotation
SBS	sphenobasilar synchondrosis
SCM	sternocleidomastoid
SD	somatic dysfunction
SI	sacroiliac
SOAP	subjective, objective, assessment, plan
SOB	shortness of breath
SP	standardized patient
ST	soft tissue
TL	thoracolumbar
TMJ	temporal mandibular joint
URI	upper respiratory infection
US	ultrasound
UTI	urinary tract infection
VS	viscerosomatic
VSR	viscerosomatic reflex(es)

INDEX

CPSIA information can be obtained
at www.ICGtesting.com
Printed in the USA
FSOW02n1503270416
19764FS